The Edge of Silence

Foreword

In the intricate and ever-evolving world of medical science, there are stories of perseverance, innovation, and unyielding hope. "The Edge of Silence" is one such story. It chronicles the journey of Dr. Alexander Carter and his dedicated team as they navigate the complexities of neurological research, driven by a relentless commitment to improve the lives of patients worldwide.

From the initial sparks of inspiration to the groundbreaking discoveries, this book offers a glimpse into the highs and lows of scientific exploration. It celebrates the power of collaboration, the strength of friendships, and the transformative impact of dedication and resilience.

As you turn these pages, you will witness the challenges faced by the team, the moments of doubt, and the ultimate triumphs that redefine the boundaries of medical science. This is not just a tale of scientific achievement; it is a testament to the human spirit and the enduring quest for knowledge and healing.

May this story inspire future generations of researchers, reminding them that with determination and hope, they too can push the edge of silence and make a lasting difference in the world.

Gal Whisby

Table of Contents

1. The Spark of an Idea
2. A New Beginning
3. Uncharted Territories
4. The First Challenge
5. Unexpected Alliances
6. Breakthroughs and Setbacks
7. Building Momentum
8. Facing Adversity
9. The Turning Point
10. Strengthening Bonds
11. Navigating Complexities
12. New Horizons
13. A Beacon of Hope
14. Overcoming Doubt
15. A Step Forward
16. Collaboration and Innovation
17. The Power of Perseverance
18. Transformative Discoveries
19. The Final Push
20. Triumph and New Beginnings
21. Reflections and Future Paths
22. Challenges Ahead
23. Breaking Barriers
24. The Pinnacle of Achievement
25. The Legacy Continues
26. Embracing the Future
27. The Uncharted Path
28. Resolute Determination
29. A Vision for Tomorrow
30. The Journey Continues
31. A Legacy of Hope

Chapter 1: The Arrival

Alex stood at the gates of MedTech University, the towering buildings casting long shadows in the late afternoon sun. The prestigious institution, known for producing some of the finest medical professionals in the country, was now his home for the next few years. He felt a mix of excitement and apprehension as he looked around, taking in the bustling campus filled with students who seemed just as eager and nervous as he was.

The journey to MedTech had been anything but easy. Alex had always been the top of his class, driven by a deep desire to help others and a promise he made to his mother before she passed away. But the pressure to succeed had taken its toll, and he often found himself wrestling with doubts about his own abilities.

With a deep breath, Alex made his way to the administration building to finalize his registration. The hallways were crowded with students, each with their own stories and struggles. As he waited in line, he couldn't help but overhear snippets of conversations—discussions about summer internships, upcoming exams, and the inevitable stress that came with being a medical student.

Finally, it was his turn. The registrar, a stern-looking woman with glasses perched on the tip of her nose, handed him a thick packet of papers. "Welcome to MedTech, Mr. Carter," she said without looking up. "You'll find all the information you need in there. Your dorm assignment, class schedule, and a map of the campus. Orientation starts tomorrow at 8 AM sharp. Don't be late."

"Thank you," Alex replied, taking the packet and making his way out of the building. He glanced at the map, trying to find his way to the dormitory. The campus was vast, and it was easy to feel overwhelmed by its size and grandeur.

As he walked, Alex couldn't shake the feeling of being a small fish in a very large pond. MedTech was known for its rigorous curriculum and high expectations, and he knew he would have to push himself harder than ever before. But beneath the anxiety, there was also a spark of determination. This was his chance to prove himself, to honor his mother's memory, and to make a difference in the world.

His dormitory, Cedar Hall, was a brick building with ivy creeping up its walls. The inside was a maze of narrow hallways and identical doors. After a few wrong turns, Alex finally found his room—number 214. He unlocked the door and stepped inside, greeted by the sight of his new roommate unpacking his bags.

"Hey, you must be Alex," the roommate said, looking up with a friendly smile. "I'm Sam. Nice to meet you."

"Nice to meet you too," Alex replied, relieved to see a friendly face. "How are you finding it here so far?"

"It's a bit overwhelming, to be honest," Sam admitted. "But I guess we'll get used to it. Everyone's in the same boat, right?"

"Yeah, I suppose so," Alex said, setting his bags down on the empty bed. The room was small but cozy, with two twin beds, a pair of desks, and a shared closet. Posters of medical anatomy and motivational quotes covered the walls, a testament to the intensity and passion of its previous occupants.

As they unpacked and settled in, Alex and Sam talked about their backgrounds, their hopes, and their fears. Sam was from a small town in the Midwest and had always dreamed of becoming a surgeon. He was easygoing and optimistic, a stark contrast to Alex's more reserved and introspective nature.

The next morning, they attended the orientation together. The auditorium was packed with first-year students, all eager to begin their journey. The dean, Dr. Thompson, gave an inspiring speech about the importance of perseverance, empathy, and dedication in the medical profession. "You are the future of medicine," he declared. "The challenges you will face here are not meant to break you but to build you into the best doctors you can be."

After the orientation, Alex and Sam explored the campus, familiarizing themselves with the lecture halls, labs, and library. Everywhere they went, they saw students immersed in their studies, some huddled in groups discussing complex medical cases, others poring over thick textbooks.

In the weeks that followed, Alex's days were filled with lectures, practical labs, and endless hours of studying. The workload was intense, and the pressure to perform was ever-present. He found solace in his friendship with Sam and the support of Dr. Matthews, a compassionate and wise professor who took a particular interest in Alex's progress.

Despite the challenges, Alex felt a growing sense of purpose. He was here for a reason, and he was determined to succeed. But as the semester progressed, he would soon realize that the path to becoming a doctor was fraught with obstacles, both external and internal, that would test his resolve in ways he never imagined.

Chapter 2: First Impressions

The morning sun filtered through the thin curtains of room 214, casting a soft glow on Alex's face. He blinked awake, momentarily disoriented, before the reality of his new life at MedTech University set in. Today marked the beginning of his first full day of classes, and with it, the first real test of his ability to keep up with the rigorous demands of medical school.

Sam was already up, flipping through a textbook at his desk. "Morning, Alex. Ready for the big day?"

Alex stretched and rubbed his eyes. "As ready as I'll ever be, I guess. What's our first class?"

"Anatomy with Dr. Whitaker. It's supposed to be one of the toughest courses in the first year," Sam replied, a hint of anxiety in his voice.

"Great," Alex muttered sarcastically. He quickly dressed and grabbed his bag, making sure to pack all the necessary textbooks and notes. As they headed out the door, Alex felt a knot of nervous energy tighten in his stomach. He had always been a diligent student, but the stakes felt much higher here.

The anatomy lecture hall was already half-full when they arrived. Students chatted quietly, reviewing notes and speculating about the difficulty of the upcoming classes. Alex and Sam found seats near the middle, giving them a good view of the front while remaining inconspicuous.

Dr. Whitaker, a tall man with a stern expression and graying hair, entered the room with a purposeful stride. He wasted no time in beginning the lecture, diving straight into a detailed overview of the human skeletal system. His rapid-fire delivery and the sheer volume of information were overwhelming, and Alex found himself struggling to keep up with his notes.

As the lecture progressed, Alex noticed a student a few rows ahead who seemed unfazed by the intensity. She was taking notes with a calm, focused demeanor, occasionally glancing up to make eye contact with Dr. Whitaker. Her confidence was impressive, and Alex felt a pang of envy.

After the lecture, Alex and Sam headed to their next class, biochemistry. As they walked, they discussed the material from anatomy, trying to reinforce what they had just learned. The campus was buzzing with activity, and everywhere they looked, students were engaged in animated conversations about their studies.

In biochemistry, they were introduced to Dr. Nguyen, a petite woman with an infectious enthusiasm for her subject. Her lecture was equally challenging but delivered with a warmth that made the complex concepts slightly more digestible. Alex found himself feeling a bit more at ease, appreciating the contrast in teaching styles.

During a break between classes, Alex and Sam grabbed coffee at the campus café. The aroma of freshly brewed coffee mingled with the chatter of students, creating a lively atmosphere. As they sipped their drinks, they were joined by another first-year student, Emily, who had been sitting near them in anatomy.

"Hey, mind if I join you?" Emily asked with a friendly smile.

"Not at all," Sam replied, motioning to an empty chair. "We were just trying to wrap our heads around Dr. Whitaker's lecture."

"Yeah, he doesn't pull any punches," Emily said, shaking her head. "But I've heard he's one of the best. I'm Emily, by the way."

"Alex," he introduced himself. "And this is Sam. How are you finding it so far?"

"It's intense," Emily admitted. "But I think we'll manage if we stick together. Study groups and all that."

"Good idea," Sam agreed. "We should definitely form a study group. Safety in numbers, right?"

As they continued to talk, Alex felt a growing sense of camaraderie. Emily was sharp and insightful, and her positive attitude was infectious. The idea of facing the challenges of MedTech with a supportive group of peers was comforting.

The rest of the day passed in a blur of lectures, lab sessions, and hurried note-taking. By the time Alex returned to his dorm room, he was exhausted but also exhilarated. The first day had been a whirlwind, but he had survived it, and he felt a small sense of accomplishment.

As he lay in bed that night, Alex thought about the road ahead. There would be many more days like this, filled with challenges and uncertainties. But he also knew he wasn't alone. With friends like Sam and Emily, and the guidance of professors like Dr. Whitaker and Dr. Nguyen, he felt a renewed determination to succeed.

And so, with a mixture of exhaustion and anticipation, Alex drifted off to sleep, ready to face whatever the next day would bring.

Chapter 3: The Pressure Mounts

The weeks following Alex's arrival at MedTech University passed in a blur of relentless study and mounting pressure. Each day, the demands grew heavier, the expectations higher. Alex found himself caught in a cycle of lectures, labs, and late-night study sessions, with little time to catch his breath.

The anatomy lab became a second home. Dr. Whitaker's intense lectures were matched by the hands-on dissections and practical exams that left little room for error. The skeletal system had been only the beginning; now, they were delving into the complexities of muscles, nerves, and organs. The sheer volume of information was overwhelming, and Alex often felt like he was drowning in it.

Sam and Emily were his lifelines, their study group becoming a sanctuary where they could share notes, quiz each other, and commiserate over the challenges they faced. Despite the support, Alex couldn't shake the growing sense of inadequacy. He had always been the top student, but here, among the best of the best, he felt painfully average.

One evening, as Alex and Sam were reviewing their notes for an upcoming exam, Sam noticed the dark circles under Alex's eyes. "You look exhausted, man. Are you getting any sleep?"

"Not much," Alex admitted. "There's just so much to cover, and I feel like I'm falling behind."

Sam nodded sympathetically. "We're all feeling the pressure, but you've got to take care of yourself too. Burning out won't help anyone."

Alex knew Sam was right, but the fear of failure kept him pushing forward. He couldn't afford to fall behind, not with everything riding on his success here.

Meanwhile, Emily seemed to be thriving, her calm demeanor and sharp intellect shining through in every class. Alex admired her ability to stay composed under pressure, and he often found himself turning to her for guidance. Emily's presence was a steadying force, and her insights helped him navigate the labyrinth of medical knowledge they were expected to master.

But not everyone was as supportive. Jessica, a fiercely competitive student, had made it clear from the start that she viewed Alex as a rival. She was brilliant, no doubt about it, but her ambition often manifested in ruthless tactics. Whether it was monopolizing the professor's time with endless questions or subtly undermining her peers, Jessica seemed determined to outshine everyone, no matter the cost.

One particularly grueling day, after hours of dissection and a challenging biochemistry lecture, Alex found a note slipped under his door. It was from Dr. Matthews, requesting a meeting. Alex's heart sank, fearing the worst. Had he done something wrong? Was he falling behind even more than he realized?

He arrived at Dr. Matthews' office, anxiety gnawing at him. The professor greeted him with a warm smile, motioning for him to sit down. "Alex, I've been watching your progress, and I can see you're struggling."

Alex felt a lump form in his throat. "I'm trying my best, but it's just so overwhelming."

Dr. Matthews nodded. "MedTech is designed to be challenging, but I believe in your potential. You're here because you have what it takes, but you need to find a balance. It's not just about working hard; it's about working smart."

He handed Alex a small book. "This helped me when I was in your shoes. It's about managing stress and finding focus. Take some time to read it. And remember, you're not alone. Reach out if you need help."

Grateful for the advice, Alex left the office feeling a glimmer of hope. He knew he had to find a way to manage the pressure if he was going to survive MedTech.

In the following days, Alex made a conscious effort to apply Dr.

Matthews' advice. He set a more structured study schedule, allowing time for breaks and relaxation. He also started attending therapy sessions offered by the university, something he had been reluctant to do at first but soon found incredibly beneficial.

Despite the improvements, the pressure continued to mount. Practical exams loomed on the horizon, each one a make-or-break moment in their academic journey. The weight of expectations from his family, his professors, and most of all, himself, bore down on Alex, a constant reminder of what was at stake.

One evening, as he sat in the library poring over histology slides, Emily joined him. "You're really pushing yourself," she observed, concern in her eyes.

"I have to," Alex replied. "There's no other way."

"There is," she insisted gently. "You're not in this alone, Alex. We're all feeling it. Lean on us. Let's get through this together."

Her words resonated with him. Alex realized that he didn't have to carry the burden by himself. With friends like Emily and Sam, and the support of mentors like Dr. Matthews, he had a network to rely on. It didn't make the journey any less challenging, but it made it more bearable.

As the semester progressed, Alex found a fragile equilibrium. He wasn't perfect, and there were still days when the pressure seemed insurmountable. But he was learning to navigate the demands of MedTech, one step at a time. And in that process, he was discovering a resilience within himself that he hadn't known existed.

Chapter 4: Secrets Unveiled

The autumn leaves had turned a brilliant shade of red and gold, creating a picturesque backdrop against the towering buildings of MedTech University. Alex walked briskly across the campus, his mind buzzing with the complexities of the upcoming exams and the mounting pressure that seemed to shadow his every step.

Despite the support of Sam and Emily, Alex couldn't shake the feeling that he was treading water, barely keeping his head above the surface. The weight of his past, the promise he had made to his mother, and the relentless competition were constant reminders of the high stakes he faced.

One evening, after a particularly grueling anatomy lab session, Alex returned to his dorm room feeling utterly drained. He dropped his backpack on the floor and collapsed onto his bed, staring at the ceiling. His mind wandered back to the last conversation he had with his mother before she passed away. Her words echoed in his mind, a blend of hope and expectation that had driven him to MedTech but now felt like a heavy burden.

The door creaked open, and Sam walked in, a concerned look on his face. "You alright, Alex? You seem out of it."

"I'm just tired," Alex replied, forcing a weak smile. "It's been a long day."

"Tell me about it," Sam said, sitting on the edge of his bed. "But you know, if you ever need to talk, I'm here."

"Thanks, Sam. I appreciate it," Alex said, grateful for his friend's unwavering support.

The next morning, Alex received a message from Dr. Matthews, asking him to come by his office. His stomach churned with anxiety as he made his way there, wondering what the professor wanted to discuss. Had he fallen behind in his studies? Was he in trouble?

Dr. Matthews greeted him with a warm smile, gesturing for him to take a seat. "Alex, I've been keeping an eye on your progress, and I wanted to check in with you. How are you holding up?"

"I'm managing," Alex replied cautiously. "It's just... a lot."

Dr. Matthews nodded. "I understand. MedTech is a challenging environment, and it's easy to feel overwhelmed. But I've noticed something about you, Alex. You have a drive that goes beyond just wanting to succeed. What's pushing you?"

Alex hesitated, unsure of how much to reveal. But there was something about Dr. Matthews' genuine concern that made him open up. "It's my mom," he began, his voice trembling slightly. "She passed away a few years ago. She always believed in me, and I promised her I would become a doctor. It's been my motivation, but sometimes it feels like too much."

Dr. Matthews listened intently, his expression softening with understanding. "I'm sorry for your loss, Alex. It's clear that your mother meant a great deal to you, and that promise is a powerful motivator. But it's also important to take care of yourself. You can't pour from an empty cup."

Alex nodded, feeling a mix of relief and sadness. "I know. It's just hard to balance everything."

"You're not alone," Dr. Matthews said gently. "Everyone here is dealing with their own struggles. And it's okay to ask for help. Have you thought about joining a support group or talking to a counselor?"

"I've been seeing a therapist," Alex admitted. "It helps, but I still feel like I'm constantly on edge."

"That's a good step," Dr. Matthews said. "Remember, it's a journey, not a race. And you're doing better than you think. If you ever need to talk, my door is always open."

After the meeting, Alex felt a weight lift from his shoulders. Dr. Matthews' words resonated with him, and he realized he wasn't alone in his struggles. There were people who cared and were willing to help him navigate the challenges of MedTech.

As the semester continued, Alex began to notice subtle changes in his approach. He still worked hard, but he also made time for self-care and reflection. His therapy sessions became a cornerstone of his routine, helping him to process his emotions and manage the stress.

One evening, as Alex was leaving the library, he bumped into Jessica. She looked flustered, her usual confident demeanor replaced by a hint of vulnerability.

"Hey, Jessica. Everything alright?" Alex asked, surprised by the unexpected encounter.

Jessica hesitated, then sighed. "Honestly, no. It's been a rough week."

Alex was taken aback by her candidness. He had always seen her as a fierce competitor, but in this moment, she seemed just as human as everyone else. "Do you want to talk about it?"

Jessica glanced around, then nodded. "Sure. Let's go for a walk."

As they strolled through the campus, Jessica opened up about the pressures she faced. "I know I come across as tough and ambitious, but it's because I have to be. My family's counting on me to succeed, and I can't afford to fail."

Alex listened, realizing that beneath her competitive exterior, Jessica was struggling with her own fears and insecurities. "I get it. We all have our reasons for being here, and the pressure can be overwhelming."

They talked for a while, sharing their experiences and fears. It was a moment of connection that shifted Alex's perception of Jessica. She wasn't just a rival; she was a fellow student navigating the same challenges.

In the weeks that followed, their relationship shifted from rivalry to mutual respect. They still competed, but there was an underlying understanding that they were all in this together, each facing their own battles.

As the semester drew to a close, Alex reflected on the journey so far. He had uncovered secrets about himself and others, realizing that everyone at MedTech carried their own burdens. It was a revelation that brought a sense of solidarity and hope, reminding him that he wasn't alone.

And so, with a renewed sense of purpose, Alex faced the challenges ahead, ready to embrace the journey with resilience and determination.

Chapter 5: The Breaking Point

The winter chill had settled over MedTech University, the once vibrant campus now blanketed in a layer of frost. Alex found himself braving the cold winds as he hurried between classes, his thoughts consumed by the upcoming practical exams. The pressure had reached an all-time high, and it seemed that every student was teetering on the edge of their endurance.

Despite his best efforts, Alex couldn't shake the growing sense of dread that followed him. His days were filled with endless lectures, lab sessions, and late-night study marathons. Sleep had become a luxury, and the weight of his promise to his mother felt heavier than ever.

One particularly brutal day, Alex faced a series of setbacks. The morning began with a difficult anatomy practical that left him second-guessing his answers. This was followed by a biochemistry quiz where his mind went blank on key concepts he had spent hours studying the night before. By the time he reached his final class of the day, he felt completely drained.

As he sat in the lecture hall, struggling to stay focused, a familiar feeling of panic began to creep in. His chest tightened, and his vision blurred. It was a panic attack, something he hadn't experienced in months. Desperate to avoid a scene, Alex gathered his belongings and rushed out of the room, barely making it to the restroom before collapsing against the wall, struggling to breathe.

After what felt like an eternity, the panic subsided, leaving him feeling weak and vulnerable. He knew he couldn't continue like this, pushing himself to the brink without regard for his own well-being. Something had to change.

That evening, as Alex sat in his dorm room staring blankly at his textbooks, Sam and Emily entered, their faces etched with concern. "We heard what happened today," Emily said softly. "Are you okay?"

"I'm fine," Alex replied automatically, but his voice lacked conviction.

"No, you're not," Sam countered. "You've been pushing yourself too hard. We're all under pressure, but you don't have to do this alone."

Emily nodded in agreement. "We need to talk to Dr. Matthews. He can help."

Reluctantly, Alex agreed. The next day, the three friends met with Dr. Matthews in his office. The professor listened intently as Alex described the panic attack and the overwhelming stress he had been under. "Alex, I'm glad you came to me," Dr. Matthews said gently. "You're facing a lot right now, and it's important to take care of your mental health."

He suggested a reduced course load for the remainder of the semester and recommended that Alex continue his therapy sessions more frequently. "There's no shame in needing help," Dr. Matthews added. "You're a talented student, and you have a bright future ahead of you. But you need to be kind to yourself."

With the support of his friends and the guidance of Dr. Matthews, Alex began to make changes. He cut back on his extracurricular activities and allowed himself more time to rest. He also opened up more during his therapy sessions, confronting the fears and anxieties that had been weighing him down.

As the weeks passed, Alex slowly began to regain his footing. The panic attacks became less frequent, and he found himself better able to manage the stress. The practical exams loomed ever closer, but he faced them with a renewed sense of determination.

The night before the anatomy practical, Alex sat in the study lounge with Sam and Emily, reviewing their notes one last time. The atmosphere was tense but supportive, each of them drawing strength from the others. "We've got this," Emily said confidently. "We've prepared as much as we can. Now we just need to trust ourselves."

The next morning, Alex entered the exam room with a mixture of anxiety and resolve. The practical was as challenging as he had anticipated, but he focused on each task with a clear mind, methodically working through the questions and procedures. When it was over, he felt a cautious sense of relief.

In the days that followed, the results of the practical were posted. Alex hesitated before looking at his score, his heart pounding. When he finally saw his results, he felt a wave of emotions wash over him. He had passed—not with top marks, but with a solid, respectable score. It was enough.

As he walked out of the exam hall, he was met by Sam and Emily, who had been waiting anxiously. "How did it go?" Sam asked.

"I passed," Alex said, a genuine smile spreading across his face for the first time in weeks.

"That's great!" Emily exclaimed, pulling him into a hug. "We knew you could do it."

The relief and joy of that moment were a stark contrast to the darkness that had threatened to consume him. Alex realized that he didn't have to be perfect; he just had to keep moving forward, one step at a time.

The semester drew to a close, and as Alex prepared to head home for the winter break, he reflected on the journey so far. It had been a tumultuous ride, filled with highs and lows, but he had learned valuable lessons about resilience, friendship, and the importance of self-care.

As he boarded the train back to his hometown, Alex felt a renewed sense of hope. The road ahead would still be challenging, but he was no longer facing it alone. With the support of his friends, mentors, and the memory of his mother guiding him, he knew he could overcome whatever obstacles lay ahead.

Chapter 6: Shadows of Doubt

The winter break had given Alex some much-needed respite from the relentless pace of MedTech University. He returned to campus feeling refreshed, but as the new semester began, the familiar pressures quickly resurfaced. The looming shadow of doubt was never far away, and Alex found himself questioning his abilities more than ever.

Classes resumed with a renewed intensity. The curriculum became even more challenging, with complex subjects like pathology and pharmacology demanding more focus and comprehension. Alex spent countless hours in the library, poring over textbooks and research papers, his mind racing to absorb the intricate details.

Despite his best efforts, Alex struggled to keep up. The material was dense, and he often found himself lost in a sea of unfamiliar terms and concepts. His confidence began to waver, and the doubts that had once been fleeting now seemed to take root in his mind.

One afternoon, during a particularly challenging pathology lecture, Alex felt his concentration slipping. Dr. Patel, a brilliant but demanding professor, was explaining the intricacies of cellular abnormalities, but Alex's mind wandered. He glanced around the lecture hall, noticing that many of his peers seemed equally perplexed.

After the lecture, Emily caught up with him. "That was intense, huh?"

"Yeah," Alex replied, trying to mask his frustration. "I feel like I'm missing something. It's all so overwhelming."

Emily nodded sympathetically. "It's a lot to take in, but we can figure it out together. How about a study session tonight? We can go over the lecture and try to make sense of it."

"That sounds good," Alex agreed, grateful for her support.

That evening, Alex, Emily, and Sam gathered in the study lounge, their notes and textbooks spread out before them. They worked through the material slowly, discussing and debating each point. Emily's calm and methodical approach helped clarify some of the more confusing aspects, while Sam's enthusiasm provided much-needed motivation.

As the hours passed, Alex began to feel a little more confident. The study session reminded him that he wasn't alone in his struggles and that together, they could tackle even the most daunting challenges.

However, the shadow of doubt continued to linger. The following week, during a pharmacology quiz, Alex found himself staring blankly at the questions. His mind went completely blank, and he struggled to recall even the most basic information. Panic set in, and he barely managed to finish the quiz before time was up.

When the results were posted, Alex's heart sank. His score was far below what he had hoped for, and the realization hit him hard. He felt a deep sense of failure and inadequacy, as if all his efforts had been in vain.

Dr. Matthews noticed Alex's distress and called him in for a meeting. "Alex, I've seen your quiz results, and I can tell you're having a tough time. What's going on?"

"I don't know," Alex admitted, his voice tinged with frustration. "I study hard, but when it comes to the tests, my mind just goes blank. I feel like I'm not good enough."

Dr. Matthews listened carefully, his expression thoughtful. "It's not uncommon to feel this way, especially in such a demanding environment. But remember, your worth isn't defined by a single quiz. You're here because you have potential, and you need to believe in that."

"But what if I'm not cut out for this?" Alex asked, voicing his deepest fear.

Dr. Matthews leaned forward, his gaze steady. "Everyone has moments of doubt, Alex. The key is to push through them and keep going. You have the ability, but you also need to have faith in yourself. Let's work on some strategies to help you manage the stress and improve your test performance."

With Dr. Matthews' guidance, Alex began to implement new study techniques and coping strategies. He focused on breaking down complex material into manageable chunks, using visualization and mnemonic devices to aid his memory. He also practiced mindfulness exercises to calm his mind and reduce anxiety before exams.

As the weeks went by, Alex slowly started to see improvements. His quiz scores began to rise, and he felt more in control during lectures and study sessions. The shadow of doubt still lingered, but it no longer paralyzed him. Instead, it served as a reminder to stay vigilant and keep pushing forward.

One evening, after a particularly successful study session, Alex sat with Sam and Emily in the cafeteria, reflecting on their journey. "It's been a rough ride, but I think we're starting to get the hang of it," Sam said, a hint of pride in his voice.

"Yeah, we are," Alex agreed. "And it's thanks to both of you. I don't think I could have made it this far without your support."

Emily smiled warmly. "We're in this together, Alex. And we're going to keep pushing each other until we reach the finish line."

As they shared a moment of camaraderie, Alex felt a renewed sense of hope. The doubts and fears that had once threatened to consume him were still there, but they were no longer insurmountable. With the support of his friends and mentors, he knew he could face whatever challenges lay ahead.

And so, with a mixture of determination and resilience, Alex continued his journey at MedTech University, ready to confront the shadows of doubt and emerge stronger on the other side.

Chapter 7: A Ray of Hope

Spring arrived at MedTech University, bringing with it a sense of renewal and fresh beginnings. The campus, once blanketed in snow, now burst with vibrant colors as flowers bloomed and trees regained their leaves. Alex felt a renewed sense of energy as he walked to class, determined to make the most of the remaining semester.

Despite the challenges of the previous months, Alex had found a rhythm that worked for him. His study sessions with Sam and Emily were more productive than ever, and the strategies he had learned from Dr. Matthews were paying off. While the shadow of doubt still lingered, it was no longer an insurmountable obstacle.

One afternoon, as Alex sat in the student lounge reviewing his notes, Dr. Matthews approached him with a thoughtful expression. "Alex, do you have a moment?"

"Of course, Dr. Matthews," Alex replied, setting his notes aside.

"I've been impressed with your progress," Dr. Matthews began. "You've shown resilience and determination, and I think you're ready for a new challenge."

Alex's curiosity was piqued. "What kind of challenge?"

Dr. Matthews handed him a brochure. "There's a summer research program at St. Vincent's Hospital. It's highly competitive, but I believe you have what it takes. It would be an excellent opportunity to apply what you've learned and gain valuable experience."

Alex scanned the brochure, excitement bubbling up inside him. The program offered hands-on research experience in a variety of medical fields, working alongside some of the best professionals in the industry. It was an opportunity he couldn't pass up.

"Thank you, Dr. Matthews. I'll definitely apply," Alex said, feeling a surge of motivation.

"Good," Dr. Matthews replied with a smile. "I think you'll do great. Just remember to take care of yourself and maintain that balance you've worked so hard to achieve."

As Alex prepared his application, he couldn't help but feel a sense of optimism. The research program represented a ray of hope, a chance to prove himself and take a significant step toward his goals. He shared the news with Sam and Emily, who were equally excited for him.

"That's amazing, Alex!" Emily exclaimed. "You'll do great. And who knows, maybe this will open even more doors for you."

"Yeah, man," Sam added. "We're proud of you."

With the support of his friends and mentors, Alex submitted his application and focused on finishing the semester strong. The final exams were demanding, but he approached them with a newfound confidence, applying the study techniques and stress management strategies that had helped him so far.

A few weeks later, as Alex was packing up his dorm room for the summer break, he received an email notification. His heart raced as he opened it, revealing the results of his application to the research program.

"Congratulations, Alex Carter," the email began. "We are pleased to inform you that you have been accepted into the St. Vincent's Hospital Summer Research Program."

Alex let out a triumphant shout, causing Sam and Emily to rush into the room. "I got in!" he exclaimed, showing them the email.

"That's awesome, Alex!" Sam said, giving him a high-five. "We knew you could do it."

Emily hugged him, beaming with pride. "This is just the beginning, Alex. You're going to do great things."

As the summer approached, Alex felt a sense of accomplishment and anticipation. The research program was a significant milestone, but it also represented a new chapter in his journey. He was eager to learn, grow, and make the most of the opportunity.

Arriving at St. Vincent's Hospital, Alex was immediately struck by the atmosphere of innovation and collaboration. The research team was composed of brilliant minds from various medical fields, each dedicated to pushing the boundaries of knowledge and improving patient care.

Under the mentorship of Dr. Harris, a renowned researcher in oncology, Alex was assigned to a project exploring new treatment methods for cancer. The work was challenging but incredibly rewarding, and Alex threw himself into it with passion and determination.

Throughout the summer, Alex experienced a series of breakthroughs and setbacks, each teaching him valuable lessons about perseverance, teamwork, and the importance of compassion in medicine. He formed strong bonds with his colleagues, who shared his dedication and drive.

One day, while reviewing data with Dr. Harris, Alex stumbled upon a promising lead. "Dr. Harris, take a look at this. The data suggests that this new compound could potentially target cancer cells more effectively than the current treatments."

Dr. Harris examined the findings, a smile spreading across his face. "Excellent work, Alex. This could be a significant breakthrough. Let's dig deeper and see where it leads."

The following weeks were a whirlwind of experiments, analysis, and late-night discussions. The team's hard work paid off, resulting in a promising new approach to cancer treatment that showed great potential in preliminary trials.

As the summer research program came to an end, Alex reflected on the incredible journey he had undertaken. The experience had not only deepened his knowledge and skills but also reinforced his commitment to making a difference in the world of medicine.

Returning to MedTech for the new semester, Alex felt a renewed sense of purpose and confidence. The ray of hope that had emerged with the research program had blossomed into a beacon, guiding him forward. With the support of his friends, mentors, and the memory of his mother, he was ready to face whatever challenges lay ahead.

Chapter 8: The Rivalry Intensifies

The start of the new semester at MedTech University brought with it a sense of renewed energy and determination. Alex returned from his summer research program at St. Vincent's Hospital with a newfound confidence and a wealth of knowledge. However, the challenges that lay ahead would test him in ways he had never imagined.

As the semester began, Alex noticed a palpable tension in the air. The competition among students had intensified, with everyone striving to excel in their courses and secure coveted internships and research opportunities. Among them, Jessica stood out as a formidable rival. Her relentless drive and ambition were well-known, and she seemed more determined than ever to come out on top.

One afternoon, during a particularly demanding pharmacology lecture, Dr. Patel announced a major project that would count for a significant portion of their grade. The project required students to work in pairs to develop a comprehensive research proposal on a cutting-edge topic in pharmacology.

As soon as the lecture ended, students scrambled to find partners. Alex immediately thought of Emily and Sam, but before he could speak to them, Jessica approached him with a confident smile. "Alex, we should team up for the project. With our combined experience, we could create something truly impressive."

Alex hesitated. He knew Jessica was brilliant, but her competitive nature made him wary. However, he couldn't deny the potential benefits of working with her. "Alright, let's do it," he agreed, hoping the collaboration would be beneficial for both of them.

Working with Jessica proved to be a double-edged sword. Her knowledge and skills were undeniably impressive, and their project quickly took shape. However, her demanding nature and relentless pursuit of perfection often led to tension. She was unyielding in her expectations, pushing Alex to his limits and beyond.

One evening, as they worked late in the library, Jessica's frustration boiled over. "Alex, you need to focus. This section isn't detailed enough. We can't afford any mistakes."

"I'm doing my best, Jessica," Alex replied, trying to keep his composure. "But we're running out of time. We need to finalize our proposal."

"Your best isn't good enough," she snapped. "We need to be exceptional if we want to stand out."

Alex took a deep breath, reminding himself that he had faced tougher challenges before. "Look, we're both tired and stressed. Let's take a break and come back to it with fresh eyes."

Jessica reluctantly agreed, and they called it a night. As Alex walked back to his dorm, he felt a mix of frustration and determination. He knew he couldn't let Jessica's intensity derail him. He had to stay focused and balanced, even in the face of mounting pressure.

The next day, Alex confided in Emily and Sam about the difficulties he was facing. "Jessica's pushing me to the brink. I don't know how much longer I can keep up with her."

"You're not alone, Alex," Emily said, her voice filled with concern. "We're here for you. If you need help, just ask."

"Yeah, man," Sam added. "Don't let her get to you. You've got this."

Their support gave Alex the strength he needed to persevere. He redoubled his efforts, balancing Jessica's demands with his own well-being. He made sure to take breaks, practice mindfulness, and rely on his friends for support.

As the deadline for the project approached, the tension between Alex and Jessica reached a boiling point. One evening, while reviewing their final draft, Jessica made a cutting remark. "If we don't get top marks, it'll be because you didn't push hard enough."

Alex had had enough. "Jessica, this isn't just about grades. It's about learning and growing. I've done my best, and I'm proud of what we've accomplished. If you can't see that, then that's on you."

Jessica was taken aback by his outburst, but she didn't respond. Instead, she silently reviewed their work, making a few final adjustments. When they finally submitted the project, Alex felt a mix of relief and exhaustion.

In the days that followed, Alex focused on his other courses and extracurricular activities, trying to regain a sense of balance. The rivalry with Jessica had taken a toll, but it had also taught him valuable lessons about resilience and self-worth.

When the project grades were finally posted, Alex was surprised to see that they had received top marks. Jessica approached him with a rare smile. "I guess we did alright after all."

"We did," Alex agreed, feeling a sense of accomplishment. "But let's not forget what's important. It's not just about winning. It's about learning and growing, together."

Jessica nodded, a thoughtful expression on her face. "Maybe you're right. Thanks for putting up with me, Alex."

As the semester continued, Alex and Jessica found a new sense of mutual respect. While their rivalry remained, it was tempered by an understanding that they were both striving for the same goal. They pushed each other to be better, but also learned to appreciate each other's strengths and weaknesses.

Alex's journey at MedTech was far from over, but he faced the challenges ahead with a renewed sense of purpose and confidence. With his friends by his side and the lessons he had learned, he knew he could overcome any obstacle.

Chapter 9: Finding Balance

The days grew longer and warmer as spring fully embraced MedTech University. With the pressures of the semester peaking, Alex found himself in a constant battle to maintain balance. The rivalry with Jessica had taught him the importance of managing stress, but the demands of his coursework and extracurricular activities still loomed large.

Despite the intense workload, Alex made a conscious effort to prioritize his well-being. He continued to practice mindfulness and took regular breaks to avoid burnout. His friends, Sam and Emily, were a constant source of support, and their study sessions provided both camaraderie and a sense of structure.

One afternoon, after a particularly grueling pharmacology lab, Emily suggested they take a break and explore a nearby park. "We need to get some fresh air and clear our heads," she said, packing up her notes.

Sam agreed. "Yeah, let's go. We've been cooped up in the library for too long."

The trio made their way to the park, where the vibrant colors of blooming flowers and the gentle rustle of leaves created a serene atmosphere. They found a quiet spot by the lake and sat down, enjoying the tranquility.

"This is exactly what we needed," Alex said, taking a deep breath. "Thanks for dragging me out here."

"No problem," Emily replied with a smile. "It's important to take breaks and recharge. We can't function at our best if we're constantly stressed."

Sam nodded. "Absolutely. We have to find a balance between work and relaxation. Otherwise, we'll burn out."

As they sat by the lake, discussing their hopes and fears, Alex felt a renewed sense of clarity. The conversation shifted from academics to personal goals and dreams, and Alex realized that his journey at

MedTech was about more than just grades and competition. It was about growth, resilience, and finding his place in the world.

The following week, Alex received an unexpected invitation from Dr. Harris, his mentor from the summer research program at St. Vincent's Hospital. Dr. Harris had been impressed with Alex's work and wanted to discuss a potential collaboration on a new project.

Excited by the opportunity, Alex met with Dr. Harris, who outlined the project's goals and scope. "We're looking at developing new treatment protocols for chronic illnesses," Dr. Harris explained. "Your insights and experience from the summer program would be invaluable."

Alex felt a surge of enthusiasm. "I'd love to be involved, Dr. Harris. This sounds like an incredible opportunity."

Dr. Harris smiled. "I knew you'd be interested. Let's get started."

Balancing his coursework with the new research project was challenging, but Alex found it invigorating. The work was demanding, but it also provided a sense of purpose and fulfillment. He was making tangible contributions to the field of medicine, and that motivated him to keep pushing forward.

Meanwhile, Alex's relationship with Jessica continued to evolve. Their rivalry had turned into a respectful partnership, and they often collaborated on projects and study sessions. Jessica's relentless drive was still present, but she had learned to temper it with a sense of teamwork and mutual support.

One evening, as they worked on a joint research paper, Jessica paused and looked at Alex. "You know, I never expected us to work so well together. I always saw you as competition, but now I see you as a valuable ally."

Alex smiled. "I felt the same way. We've both grown a lot since the beginning. I'm glad we can support each other."

Jessica nodded. "Me too. Let's make sure we continue to do that."

As the semester progressed, Alex found himself in a better place than he had been in months. He had learned to balance his academic and personal life, and his relationships with his friends and colleagues had deepened. The lessons he had learned about resilience, collaboration, and self-care were paying off, and he felt more equipped to handle whatever challenges lay ahead.

The final exams approached, bringing with them the usual stress and anxiety. However, this time Alex felt more prepared. He tackled his studies with a sense of calm determination, knowing that he had the tools and support to succeed.

On the day of the last exam, Alex entered the exam hall with a mixture of nerves and confidence. He took a deep breath, reminded himself of all the hard work he had put in, and began the test. The questions were challenging, but he methodically worked through them, applying everything he had learned.

When the exam was over, Alex felt a wave of relief and satisfaction. He had given it his all, and now it was time to wait for the results. As he left the hall, he was greeted by Sam and Emily, who had finished their exams as well.

"We did it!" Sam exclaimed, his face lighting up with a grin. "The semester's over!"

Emily nodded, her eyes shining with pride. "We made it through. Now it's time to celebrate."

They decided to celebrate their accomplishments with a dinner at their favorite restaurant. As they enjoyed their meal, they reflected on the journey they had shared and the challenges they had overcome.

"Here's to finding balance," Alex said, raising his glass. "And to the amazing friends who helped me get through it all."

"To balance and friendship," Emily agreed, clinking her glass with his.

As they celebrated, Alex felt a deep sense of gratitude. The road at MedTech had been tough, but he had grown stronger and more resilient with each step. With the support of his friends, mentors, and newfound sense of balance, he was ready to face whatever the future held.

Chapter 10: The Dark Night

The celebration of completing their final exams was short-lived. A few weeks into the new semester, Alex and his friends were thrust into a situation that would test their resilience like never before. The weather had turned unexpectedly harsh, with a relentless storm sweeping across the region, casting a literal and figurative shadow over MedTech University.

One evening, as the storm raged outside, Alex sat in his dorm room, trying to focus on his studies. The howling wind and pounding rain made it difficult to concentrate. Suddenly, his phone buzzed with a message from Emily.

"Urgent meeting in the common room. Now."

Alex felt a pang of anxiety as he hurried to the common room, where he found Sam, Emily, and several other students gathered. Their faces were etched with concern and worry.

"What's going on?" Alex asked, his voice tense.

Emily stepped forward, her expression grave. "There's been a serious accident. Dr. Matthews was in a car crash on his way home from campus. He's in critical condition at the hospital."

A stunned silence fell over the group. Dr. Matthews had been a mentor and guiding light for many of them, including Alex. The news hit hard, and Alex felt a wave of emotions—shock, fear, and a deep sense of helplessness.

"Is there anything we can do?" Sam asked, his voice breaking the silence.

"We need to be there for each other," Emily replied. "And for Dr. Matthews. We can't let this derail us. We have to stay strong."

The next few days were a blur of uncertainty and worry. Alex and his friends visited the hospital, where they were met with a somber atmosphere. Dr. Matthews lay unconscious, surrounded by medical equipment and a team of doctors fighting to stabilize him.

Seeing his mentor in such a vulnerable state was a profound shock for Alex. He had always seen Dr. Matthews as a pillar of strength and wisdom. Now, he was reminded of the fragility of life and the unpredictable nature of their journey.

As the storm continued to rage outside, Alex found solace in the support of his friends. They spent long hours in the hospital waiting room, sharing stories and memories of Dr. Matthews, finding comfort in each other's presence.

One evening, while they were gathered in the waiting room, Jessica appeared. She looked distraught, her usual confident demeanor replaced by a deep sadness.

"How is he?" she asked, her voice barely above a whisper.

"No change," Emily replied gently. "But we're hoping for the best."

Jessica sat down, her eyes filled with tears. "I can't believe this is happening. Dr. Matthews has been such an important part of our lives."

Alex placed a reassuring hand on her shoulder. "We're all in this together, Jessica. We'll get through it."

The days turned into weeks, and the storm eventually subsided. Dr. Matthews' condition remained critical, but there were small signs of improvement. The support and prayers of the students seemed to make a difference, giving them hope in the face of adversity.

During this difficult time, Alex leaned heavily on the lessons he had learned about resilience and balance. He continued to attend classes and work on his research project, finding a delicate equilibrium between his responsibilities and the emotional toll of Dr. Matthews' condition.

One night, as Alex was leaving the hospital after a long visit, he bumped into Dr. Harris, who had come to check on Dr. Matthews. They spoke briefly, and Dr. Harris offered some words of encouragement.

"You're doing great, Alex. Keep your focus and stay strong. Dr. Matthews would be proud of you."

Alex nodded, feeling a renewed sense of determination. He realized that Dr. Matthews had instilled in him the tools and mindset needed to navigate even the darkest of times.

As the semester progressed, Alex and his friends found strength in their shared experience. They continued to support each other, drawing on their collective resilience to face the challenges ahead. Dr. Matthews' situation served as a stark reminder of the unpredictability of life, but it also reinforced the importance of perseverance and hope.

One afternoon, as Alex was studying in the library, he received a text from Emily. "Come to the hospital. There's news."

Alex's heart raced as he made his way to the hospital. When he arrived, he found Emily, Sam, and Jessica gathered in the waiting room, their faces filled with cautious optimism.

"Dr. Matthews is awake," Emily said, her voice trembling with emotion. "He's not out of the woods yet, but he's conscious and responsive."

A wave of relief and joy washed over Alex. They hurried to Dr. Matthews' room, where they found him awake and smiling weakly. Though he was still frail, there was a spark in his eyes that gave them hope.

"Thank you for being here," Dr. Matthews said softly, his voice weak but filled with gratitude. "Your support means everything to me."

Tears welled up in Alex's eyes as he responded. "We're here for you, Dr. Matthews. Always."

The recovery process was slow, but Dr. Matthews gradually regained his strength. His resilience and determination served as an inspiration to everyone around him. As Alex and his friends continued their studies, they carried with them the lessons learned during this challenging time.

The dark night had tested their limits, but it had also brought them closer together and strengthened their resolve. They had faced adversity head-on and emerged stronger, with a deeper understanding of the power of hope, resilience, and the unwavering support of friends and mentors.

As the semester drew to a close, Alex felt a renewed sense of purpose. The journey ahead would undoubtedly hold more challenges, but he knew that with the strength and support of his friends, he could face anything.

Chapter 11: Rising from the Ashes

The aftermath of Dr. Matthews' accident had cast a long shadow over MedTech University, but as the new semester began, a sense of renewal slowly emerged. Dr. Matthews' gradual recovery served as a beacon of hope, reminding everyone of the resilience that defined their journey.

Alex, Emily, Sam, and Jessica found strength in their shared experiences. The ordeal had brought them closer, forging bonds that went beyond academic competition. They supported each other through the challenges, drawing on the lessons they had learned about perseverance and balance.

One morning, as the spring sun filtered through the windows of the library, Alex received an email from Dr. Matthews. The subject line read, "A New Opportunity." Curious and excited, Alex quickly opened the email.

"Dear Alex,

I hope this message finds you well. I am pleased to inform you that I have been cleared to return to teaching part-time. Your support during my recovery has been invaluable, and I am deeply grateful.

I have a new research project that I believe you would be perfect for. It focuses on developing innovative treatments for neurological disorders, a field that holds great promise and urgency. I would like you to be a part of this project, as your insights and dedication have impressed me greatly.

Please let me know if you are interested. I look forward to working with you again.

Best regards,
Dr. Matthews"

Alex's heart swelled with pride and excitement. The opportunity to work with Dr. Matthews on such a groundbreaking project was a dream come true. He immediately replied, expressing his enthusiasm and gratitude.

Later that day, Alex shared the news with his friends. "Dr. Matthews is back, and he's invited me to join his new research project on neurological disorders!"

"That's amazing, Alex!" Emily exclaimed, her eyes sparkling with pride. "You deserve it."

Sam clapped him on the back. "You're going to do great things, man. We always knew it."

Jessica nodded, a rare smile on her face. "Congratulations, Alex. This is a big step forward."

The new research project demanded Alex's full attention, but he approached it with a renewed sense of purpose and determination. Dr. Matthews' guidance and mentorship were invaluable, and Alex felt privileged to be part of a team working on such critical and innovative treatments.

The project focused on exploring new approaches to treating conditions like Parkinson's disease and Alzheimer's. Alex immersed himself in the research, analyzing data, conducting experiments, and collaborating with fellow researchers. The work was challenging, but it also provided a profound sense of fulfillment.

As the weeks passed, Alex and his team made significant strides. They identified a promising compound that showed potential in slowing the progression of neurological disorders. The discovery brought a wave of excitement and optimism to the team, fueling their determination to push forward.

One evening, as Alex was reviewing data in the lab, Dr. Matthews approached him with a thoughtful expression. "Alex, I've been impressed with your dedication and insights. Your work on this project has been outstanding."

"Thank you, Dr. Matthews," Alex replied, humbled by the praise. "I couldn't have done it without your guidance."

Dr. Matthews smiled. "You're a natural leader, Alex. Have you considered presenting our findings at the upcoming medical conference?"

Alex's eyes widened in surprise. "I hadn't thought about it, but I'd be honored."

"Good," Dr. Matthews said. "I think you have a lot to offer, and this would be a great opportunity to showcase our work and your contributions."

The prospect of presenting at a major medical conference was both exhilarating and nerve-wracking. Alex spent countless hours preparing, refining his presentation, and practicing in front of his friends. Emily, Sam, and Jessica provided invaluable feedback and support, helping him hone his delivery and build his confidence.

The day of the conference arrived, and Alex felt a mixture of excitement and anxiety as he took the stage. The auditorium was filled with esteemed medical professionals, researchers, and students. As he began his presentation, he focused on the importance of their work and the potential impact on patients' lives.

As he spoke, Alex felt a surge of confidence. He highlighted the team's findings, the innovative approaches they had developed, and the promising results. The audience listened intently, and when he concluded, the room erupted in applause.

Dr. Matthews beamed with pride as he joined Alex on stage. "You did an outstanding job, Alex. I'm incredibly proud of you."

The conference proved to be a turning point in Alex's journey. The recognition and positive feedback from the medical community validated the team's hard work and reinforced the importance of their research. It also opened new doors, leading to further collaborations and opportunities.

Back at MedTech, Alex continued to balance his coursework with the demands of the research project. The support of his friends and the mentorship of Dr. Matthews fueled his determination to push the boundaries of medical science.

As the semester progressed, Alex found himself reflecting on the journey that had brought him to this point. The challenges, setbacks, and moments of doubt had all contributed to his growth and resilience. He had learned that true strength came from perseverance, collaboration, and the unwavering support of those around him.

One evening, as Alex and his friends gathered to celebrate their latest achievements, he raised his glass in a toast. "To resilience, friendship, and the pursuit of knowledge. We've come a long way, and I couldn't have done it without all of you."

"To resilience and friendship," Emily echoed, clinking her glass with his.

"And to the future," Sam added. "Whatever it holds, we're ready."

As they celebrated, Alex felt a profound sense of gratitude. The journey had been challenging, but it had also been incredibly rewarding. With the support of his friends, mentors, and the lessons he had learned, he knew that he was ready to face whatever the future held.

Chapter 12: The Turning Point

The summer sun shone brightly over MedTech University as the new semester brought with it a sense of renewal and anticipation. The research project with Dr. Matthews had been a resounding success, and Alex felt a newfound sense of confidence as he navigated his academic journey. However, the path ahead would present challenges that would test his resolve and shape his future in unexpected ways.

One morning, as Alex was preparing for his classes, he received an email from Dr. Harris, the renowned researcher he had worked with at St. Vincent's Hospital. The subject line read, "Exciting Opportunity." Intrigued, Alex quickly opened the email.

"Dear Alex,

I hope this message finds you well. I have been following your progress and am impressed with your achievements. I am currently leading a new clinical trial on innovative treatments for chronic neurological disorders, and I believe your expertise and dedication would be a valuable addition to our team.

The trial will take place at our state-of-the-art research facility, and it will involve extensive collaboration with leading experts in the field. This is a unique opportunity to contribute to groundbreaking research and make a significant impact on patient care.

Please let me know if you are interested. I look forward to the possibility of working with you again.

Best regards,
Dr. Harris"

Alex's heart raced with excitement. The opportunity to work on a clinical trial with Dr. Harris was a dream come true, but he knew it would require a significant commitment and might affect his studies at MedTech. He needed to discuss this with his friends and mentors before making a decision.

Later that day, Alex gathered with Emily, Sam, and Jessica in the campus café. He shared the email with them, eager to hear their thoughts.

"Wow, Alex, that's an incredible opportunity," Emily said, her eyes wide with excitement. "But it's also a big commitment. How do you feel about it?"

"I'm thrilled," Alex admitted. "But I'm also worried about balancing the trial with my coursework. I don't want to fall behind."

Sam nodded thoughtfully. "It's definitely a tough decision, but you've always managed to balance everything so well. If anyone can do it, it's you."

Jessica added, "And don't forget, we're here to support you. Whatever you decide, we'll help you make it work."

Encouraged by their support, Alex decided to seek Dr. Matthews' advice. He found his mentor in the research lab, engrossed in a new project.

"Dr. Matthews, do you have a moment?" Alex asked, feeling a mix of excitement and apprehension.

"Of course, Alex. What's on your mind?" Dr. Matthews replied, looking up from his work.

Alex explained the opportunity presented by Dr. Harris and his concerns about balancing the clinical trial with his studies. Dr. Matthews listened intently, his expression thoughtful.

"Alex, this is indeed a remarkable opportunity," Dr. Matthews said after a moment. "But you're right to consider the challenges it poses. Balancing a clinical trial with your coursework will be demanding, but I believe you have the capability to succeed. The key will be to manage your time effectively and prioritize your responsibilities."

He paused, then added, "I can also speak with your professors to see if any accommodations can be made to support your participation in the trial. This kind of experience is invaluable, and I believe it will greatly enhance your education and future career."

With Dr. Matthews' reassurance and support, Alex felt more confident about his decision. He replied to Dr. Harris, expressing his interest and gratitude for the opportunity. Within days, the arrangements were made, and Alex found himself embarking on a new and challenging journey.

The clinical trial was intense and demanding, requiring meticulous attention to detail and long hours of work. Alex collaborated with a team of researchers, doctors, and technicians, all dedicated to finding innovative treatments for chronic neurological disorders. The work was both exhilarating and exhausting, pushing Alex to his limits but also providing a profound sense of fulfillment.

Balancing the trial with his studies proved to be a constant challenge. There were days when Alex felt overwhelmed, but he drew strength from the support of his friends and mentors. Emily, Sam, and Jessica helped him stay on top of his coursework, often studying together late into the night.

As the weeks turned into months, the trial began to show promising results. The team's innovative treatments were making a tangible difference in the lives of patients, and the sense of accomplishment fueled Alex's determination to keep pushing forward.

One evening, as Alex was reviewing data in the lab, Dr. Harris approached him with a look of admiration. "Alex, your contributions to this trial have been outstanding. Your dedication and hard work have played a crucial role in our success."

"Thank you, Dr. Harris," Alex replied, humbled by the praise. "It's been an incredible experience, and I'm grateful for the opportunity to be part of this team."

Dr. Harris smiled. "I have no doubt that you have a bright future ahead of you. Keep up the excellent work, and remember that the journey is just as important as the destination."

The trial eventually concluded, and the results were published in a prestigious medical journal. Alex's name appeared alongside those of the leading researchers, a testament to his dedication and hard work. The recognition brought a sense of pride and validation, reinforcing his commitment to making a difference in the field of medicine.

As the semester drew to a close, Alex reflected on the journey he had undertaken. The turning point had come with challenges and sacrifices, but it had also brought growth, resilience, and a deeper understanding of his purpose. With the support of his friends, mentors, and the experiences he had gained, Alex felt more prepared than ever to face the future.

One evening, as they gathered to celebrate their achievements, Alex raised his glass in a toast. "To turning points, resilience, and the journey ahead. We've faced challenges, but we've also grown stronger and closer. Here's to whatever the future holds."

"To the future," Emily echoed, clinking her glass with his.

"And to the incredible journey we've shared," Sam added.

Jessica smiled. "We've come a long way, and I can't wait to see where we go next."

As they celebrated, Alex felt a profound sense of gratitude and anticipation. The journey was far from over, but with the support and strength of his friends and mentors, he knew that he was ready to embrace whatever lay ahead.

Chapter 13: Trials and Triumphs

The summer had transitioned into a crisp autumn, and the vibrant colors of the changing leaves painted a beautiful backdrop at MedTech University. Alex felt a sense of anticipation as he embarked on the new semester. The successes of the clinical trial had bolstered his confidence, but he knew that new challenges lay ahead.

One morning, Alex received an unexpected call from his father. "Alex, I need to talk to you about something important. Can you come home this weekend?"

Concerned by the seriousness in his father's voice, Alex agreed. He arrived home to find his father waiting for him with a solemn expression. "Dad, what's going on?" Alex asked, feeling a knot form in his stomach.

His father took a deep breath. "Alex, your mother has been diagnosed with early-stage Alzheimer's. The doctors are optimistic, but we need to start treatment right away."

The news hit Alex like a ton of bricks. He had dedicated his studies to understanding and treating neurological disorders, but now it was personal. The weight of the situation felt overwhelming, and he struggled to process the emotions swirling inside him.

"We'll get through this, Dad," Alex said, trying to reassure both himself and his father. "I've been working on treatments for this. I'll do everything I can to help Mom."

Returning to MedTech with a renewed sense of purpose, Alex threw himself into his studies and research with even greater determination. The knowledge that his work could directly impact his mother's life fueled his drive to excel.

One evening, as Alex was working late in the lab, Emily found him, concern etched on her face. "Alex, you've been pushing yourself too hard. You need to take a break."

"I can't, Emily," Alex replied, his voice tinged with frustration. "This is too important. My mom needs me."

Emily placed a comforting hand on his shoulder. "I understand, but you can't help her if you burn out. We're all here to support you, but you need to take care of yourself too."

Reluctantly, Alex agreed to take a short break. He joined Emily, Sam, and Jessica for a quiet evening in the common room, where they watched a movie and shared stories. The camaraderie and laughter provided a much-needed respite from the stress.

As the semester progressed, Alex continued to balance his coursework, research, and personal life. The support of his friends and mentors was invaluable, helping him navigate the challenges with resilience and determination.

In the midst of his busy schedule, Alex received an invitation to present his research at an international medical conference. The recognition was a significant honor, and Alex felt a surge of pride. However, the timing was difficult, as his mother's condition required ongoing attention and care.

He discussed the opportunity with Dr. Matthews, who offered his support and guidance. "Alex, this is a remarkable achievement, and I believe you should seize it. Your work has the potential to make a significant impact. We can arrange for accommodations so you can balance both your responsibilities here and the conference."

With Dr. Matthews' encouragement, Alex decided to accept the invitation. The conference was a whirlwind of presentations, discussions, and networking. Alex had the chance to meet leading experts in the field, and he shared his research with a receptive and enthusiastic audience.

During one of the sessions, Alex was approached by Dr. Elena Vasquez, a renowned neurologist known for her groundbreaking work in Alzheimer's research. "Alex, your presentation was impressive. Your approach to treatment is innovative and shows great promise. I'd like to discuss a potential collaboration."

Alex was thrilled by the prospect. "Thank you, Dr. Vasquez. I'd be honored to collaborate with you. My mother's recent diagnosis has made this work even more personal for me."

Dr. Vasquez nodded, understanding the gravity of his words. "Let's work together to make a difference. We can combine our expertise and resources to develop more effective treatments."

Returning to MedTech with new insights and collaborations, Alex felt a renewed sense of hope. The trials and triumphs of the past months had tested his limits, but they had also revealed his strength and resilience.

One evening, as he sat in the library reviewing his notes, Alex received a call from his father. "Alex, I have good news. Your mother's treatment is showing positive results. The doctors are optimistic about her progress."

Tears of relief filled Alex's eyes. "That's wonderful, Dad. I'm so glad to hear it."

As he hung up the phone, Alex felt a profound sense of gratitude. The journey had been challenging, but the support of his friends, mentors, and the breakthroughs in his research had made a tangible difference.

Gathering with Emily, Sam, and Jessica to share the good news, Alex raised his glass in a toast. "To trials and triumphs, and to the incredible support of friends and family. We've faced challenges, but we've also achieved so much. Here's to continuing this journey together."

"To friendship and perseverance," Emily echoed, clinking her glass with his.

"And to making a difference," Sam added.

Jessica smiled warmly. "We've come a long way, and I'm proud of us all."

As they celebrated, Alex felt a deep sense of fulfillment. The road ahead would undoubtedly hold more challenges, but with the strength of their bonds and the determination to make a difference, he knew they could overcome anything.

Chapter 14: Facing the Unknown

As winter descended upon MedTech University, the campus was blanketed in a crisp layer of snow. The cold air carried a sense of stillness, but within the walls of the university, a whirlwind of activity and anticipation marked the final stretch of the semester. Alex felt a mixture of excitement and trepidation as he prepared to face new challenges and uncertainties.

One morning, Alex received an urgent email from Dr. Harris. The subject line read, "Immediate Attention Required." Concerned, Alex quickly opened the email.

"Dear Alex,

I hope you are well. I regret to inform you that there has been a significant development in our ongoing clinical trial. Some unexpected complications have arisen with a subset of patients, and we need to address these issues immediately. Your expertise and insights will be crucial in navigating this situation.

Please join an emergency meeting this afternoon to discuss our next steps.

Best regards,
Dr. Harris"

Alex felt a knot of anxiety form in his stomach. The clinical trial had shown so much promise, and the thought of complications was daunting. He knew that this would be a critical moment, not just for the trial, but for his career and the patients depending on their research.

He attended the emergency meeting, where Dr. Harris outlined the complications they were facing. Some patients had developed adverse reactions to the treatment, and the team needed to determine the cause and find a solution quickly.

"Alex, your experience and dedication have been invaluable to this trial,"

Dr. Harris said. "We need your help to analyze the data and identify potential solutions."

The gravity of the situation weighed heavily on Alex, but he felt a surge of determination. "I'll do everything I can, Dr. Harris. Let's get to work."

The following weeks were a blur of long hours, intense discussions, and meticulous analysis. Alex and the research team pored over the data, conducted additional tests, and explored every possible avenue to address the complications. The pressure was immense, but the stakes were too high to falter.

One evening, as Alex was working late in the lab, Emily stopped by with a cup of coffee. "You've been at this non-stop, Alex. How are you holding up?"

"I'm exhausted, but we can't afford to stop," Alex replied, taking a grateful sip of the coffee. "These patients are counting on us."

Emily nodded, her expression filled with concern and admiration. "Just remember, you're not alone. We're all here to support you."

With the encouragement of his friends and the guidance of his mentors, Alex pushed through the challenges. The team discovered that a specific genetic marker was linked to the adverse reactions, allowing them to adjust the treatment protocol and mitigate the risks. The breakthrough brought a sense of relief and renewed hope.

Dr. Harris called a meeting to announce the findings. "Thanks to the tireless efforts of our team, we've identified the cause of the complications and implemented a solution. This is a significant achievement, and I want to commend Alex for his exceptional contributions."

The room erupted in applause, and Alex felt a wave of pride and gratitude. The journey had been arduous, but the outcome was worth every effort.

As the semester drew to a close, Alex reflected on the trials and triumphs he had faced. The experience had tested his limits, but it had also revealed his resilience and capacity for growth. With the support of his friends, mentors, and the determination to make a difference, he had navigated the unknown and emerged stronger.

One evening, as Alex and his friends gathered to celebrate the end of the semester, he raised his glass in a toast. "To facing the unknown, and to the strength and support that help us overcome any challenge. We've come a long way, and I couldn't have done it without all of you."

"To resilience and friendship," Emily echoed, clinking her glass with his.

"And to the incredible journey ahead," Sam added.

Jessica smiled warmly. "We've faced so much, and I'm proud of us all. Here's to whatever comes next."

As they celebrated, Alex felt a deep sense of fulfillment and anticipation. The future held many uncertainties, but with the strength of their bonds and the lessons they had learned, he knew they were ready to face anything together.

Chapter 15: A Glimmer of Hope

The new year dawned with a sense of renewed hope and determination at MedTech University. Alex felt the weight of the challenges he had faced in the past year, but he also carried a sense of accomplishment and growth. With the support of his friends and mentors, he was ready to embrace the opportunities and obstacles that lay ahead.

One morning, as Alex was preparing for his clinical rounds, he received a call from Dr. Vasquez. "Alex, I have some exciting news. Our collaborative research has shown promising results, and I believe we are on the verge of a significant breakthrough. I would like you to present our findings at the upcoming Global Neurology Conference."

Alex's heart raced with excitement. The opportunity to present their research on such a prestigious platform was a dream come true. "Thank you, Dr. Vasquez. I'm honored and thrilled by this opportunity."

As he prepared for the conference, Alex immersed himself in the data, refining his presentation and rehearsing his delivery. The support of his friends was invaluable, as they helped him practice and offered constructive feedback.

The day of the conference arrived, and Alex felt a mixture of nerves and excitement as he took the stage. The audience was filled with esteemed neurologists, researchers, and medical professionals from around the world. Alex began his presentation, highlighting the innovative approaches and promising results of their research.

As he spoke, Alex felt a surge of confidence. He shared the story of their journey, the challenges they had overcome, and the hope their research brought to patients suffering from neurological disorders. When he concluded, the room erupted in applause, and Alex felt a profound sense of accomplishment.

After the presentation, Dr. Vasquez approached him with a smile. "You did an outstanding job, Alex. Your passion and dedication are truly inspiring."

"Thank you, Dr. Vasquez," Alex replied, humbled by the praise. "I'm grateful for the opportunity to work with you and contribute to this important research."

The conference proved to be a turning point in Alex's career. The recognition and positive feedback from the medical community opened new doors and led to further collaborations. Alex felt a renewed sense of purpose and determination to continue making a difference in the field of neurology.

As the semester progressed, Alex balanced his coursework, research, and clinical duties with a sense of focus and resilience. The support of his friends and mentors remained a constant source of strength, helping him navigate the challenges and uncertainties.

One evening, as Alex was working late in the lab, he received a call from his father. "Alex, I have some wonderful news. Your mother's latest tests show significant improvement. The doctors are optimistic about her progress."

Tears of joy filled Alex's eyes. "That's amazing, Dad. I'm so relieved and grateful."

As he hung up the phone, Alex felt a deep sense of gratitude. The journey had been challenging, but the progress his mother had made was a testament to the importance of their work and the power of hope.

Gathering with Emily, Sam, and Jessica to share the good news, Alex raised his glass in a toast. "To hope, resilience, and the power of making a difference. We've faced many challenges, but we've also achieved so much. Here's to the incredible journey ahead."

"To hope and perseverance," Emily echoed, clinking her glass with his.

"And to the strength of our friendships," Sam added.

Jessica smiled warmly. "We've come a long way, and I'm proud of us all. Here's to the future."

As they celebrated, Alex felt a profound sense of fulfillment and anticipation. The challenges and triumphs of the past year had shaped him in ways he never imagined. With the support of his friends, mentors, and the knowledge that their work was making a tangible difference, Alex felt ready to face whatever the future held.

Chapter 16: New Horizons

Spring had arrived at MedTech University, bringing with it a sense of renewal and optimism. The campus buzzed with excitement as students prepared for graduation and the next chapters of their lives. Alex stood at a crossroads, reflecting on the journey that had brought him to this moment and contemplating the future that lay ahead.

One morning, as Alex was heading to his final clinical rounds, he received a call from Dr. Matthews. "Alex, I'd like to see you in my office this afternoon. I have something important to discuss with you."

Curiosity piqued, Alex agreed and made his way to Dr. Matthews' office later that day. He found his mentor waiting with a smile. "Alex, you've come a long way since you first arrived at MedTech. Your dedication and hard work have not gone unnoticed. I have an exciting opportunity for you."

Dr. Matthews handed Alex a brochure. "The International Institute for Neurological Research has invited you to join their team as a research fellow. This institute is at the forefront of groundbreaking neurological studies, and I believe this position would be an incredible next step for you."

Alex's eyes widened with excitement as he scanned the brochure. "This is amazing, Dr. Matthews. Thank you for believing in me."

Dr. Matthews nodded. "You've earned it, Alex. Your work has shown great promise, and I have no doubt that you'll continue to make significant contributions to the field."

As Alex considered the opportunity, he felt a mix of emotions. The chance to work at the International Institute for Neurological Research was a dream come true, but it also meant leaving behind the familiar surroundings and close friends at MedTech.

That evening, Alex shared the news with Emily, Sam, and Jessica. "I've been offered a research fellowship at the International Institute for

Neurological Research."

"Wow, Alex, that's incredible!" Emily exclaimed, her eyes shining with pride. "You deserve this."

Sam clapped him on the back. "You're going to do great things, man. We're so proud of you."

Jessica smiled warmly. "It's an amazing opportunity, Alex. We're all here to support you, no matter where you go."

As the end of the semester approached, Alex focused on wrapping up his studies and preparing for the transition. The support of his friends and mentors was invaluable, helping him navigate the bittersweet emotions of leaving MedTech and embracing the new opportunities ahead.

On the day of graduation, Alex stood with his friends, feeling a sense of pride and accomplishment. The ceremony was a celebration of their hard work, resilience, and the bonds they had formed. As they tossed their caps into the air, Alex felt a surge of optimism for the future.

In the weeks that followed, Alex prepared for his move to the International Institute for Neurological Research. The anticipation of new challenges and discoveries filled him with excitement. On his last night at MedTech, Alex and his friends gathered for a farewell dinner.

"Here's to new horizons," Alex said, raising his glass in a toast. "We've come a long way, and I couldn't have done it without all of you. Let's stay connected and continue to support each other, no matter where life takes us."

"To new horizons," Emily echoed, clinking her glass with his.

"And to the incredible journey ahead," Sam added.

Jessica smiled warmly. "We've faced so much together, and I'm excited to see what the future holds for all of us."

As they celebrated, Alex felt a profound sense of gratitude. The journey at MedTech had been transformative, shaping him into the person he was today. With the support of his friends, mentors, and the promise of new horizons, Alex was ready to embrace the future with confidence and determination.

Chapter 17: The Research Fellow

The day had finally arrived for Alex to embark on his new journey at the International Institute for Neurological Research. The bustling city around the institute contrasted sharply with the familiar surroundings of MedTech University. As he stood in front of the imposing building, Alex felt a mix of excitement and nerves. This was a new beginning, a chance to make a significant impact in the field he was passionate about.

The first few days were a whirlwind of orientation sessions, meeting new colleagues, and familiarizing himself with the state-of-the-art facilities. The institute was a hub of innovation, filled with brilliant minds dedicated to pushing the boundaries of medical science. Alex was assigned to work under Dr. Elena Vasquez, whose reputation as a leading neurologist was well-earned.

"Welcome to the team, Alex," Dr. Vasquez said warmly as they met in her office. "I've been looking forward to working with you. Your previous research has shown great promise, and I believe you'll make valuable contributions here."

"Thank you, Dr. Vasquez. I'm excited and ready to get started," Alex replied, feeling a surge of motivation.

The project they were working on focused on developing new treatments for neurodegenerative diseases. The complexity and scale of the research were daunting, but Alex thrived on the challenge. He spent long hours in the lab, analyzing data, conducting experiments, and collaborating with his colleagues.

One evening, as Alex was deep in thought, reviewing a particularly perplexing set of data, Dr. Vasquez approached him. "Alex, you've been working tirelessly. How about we take a break and grab some coffee?"

Grateful for the suggestion, Alex agreed. As they sat in the institute's café, Dr. Vasquez shared her insights and experiences. "The work we're doing here is incredibly important, but it can also be overwhelming. It's crucial to find a balance and remember why we're doing this."

Alex nodded, absorbing her wisdom. "You're right. Sometimes it's easy to get lost in the details and forget the bigger picture."

As the weeks turned into months, Alex found his rhythm. He continued to draw strength from the support of his friends, who stayed in touch regularly, offering encouragement and advice. Emily, Sam, and Jessica were all thriving in their respective paths, and their bond remained as strong as ever.

One day, while analyzing a new compound, Alex noticed something unusual. The data suggested that the compound had a unique mechanism of action that could potentially slow the progression of Alzheimer's disease more effectively than current treatments. Excited by the discovery, he immediately shared his findings with Dr. Vasquez.

"This is remarkable, Alex," Dr. Vasquez said, examining the data closely. "If this holds up in further testing, it could be a significant breakthrough."

They quickly mobilized the team to conduct additional experiments and validate the findings. The process was meticulous and required rigorous scrutiny, but the initial results were promising. The compound showed potential not only in slowing the progression but also in improving cognitive function.

As the news spread, the institute buzzed with excitement. The research attracted attention from leading experts and media outlets, eager to learn more about the potential breakthrough. Alex found himself thrust into the spotlight, giving interviews and presenting their findings at conferences.

During one such conference, Alex was approached by Dr. Richard Morgan, a prominent figure in the field of neurology. "Alex, your work is impressive. I'd like to discuss a potential collaboration that could further advance our understanding and treatment of neurodegenerative diseases."

Honored by the recognition, Alex agreed to explore the collaboration.

The opportunity to work with Dr. Morgan and his team was another step forward in his career, and he was eager to see where it would lead.

Despite the whirlwind of activity and accolades, Alex remained grounded. He never forgot the personal connection that had driven him to this field—his mother's battle with Alzheimer's. The progress she had made with her treatment was a constant reminder of the real impact their work could have on patients and families.

As the project progressed, Alex faced new challenges and setbacks, but his resilience and determination never wavered. He knew that each obstacle was an opportunity to learn and grow. The support of his colleagues and the guidance of Dr. Vasquez were invaluable, helping him navigate the complexities of their research.

One evening, as Alex was leaving the lab, Dr. Vasquez caught up with him. "Alex, I want to commend you on your dedication and perseverance. You've shown remarkable leadership and innovation. I'm confident that together, we can achieve great things."

"Thank you, Dr. Vasquez," Alex replied, feeling a deep sense of gratitude. "It's been an incredible journey, and I'm excited to see what the future holds."

As he walked through the bustling city streets, Alex reflected on the path that had brought him here. The journey from MedTech University to the International Institute for Neurological Research had been filled with challenges, triumphs, and invaluable lessons. With each step, he had grown stronger and more determined to make a difference.

With the support of his friends, mentors, and the knowledge that their work was making a tangible impact, Alex felt ready to embrace the future. The horizon was filled with possibilities, and he was eager to explore them, one breakthrough at a time.

Chapter 18: Unexpected Revelations

The progress at the International Institute for Neurological Research was both exhilarating and exhausting. Alex had settled into his role, finding a balance between the demands of groundbreaking research and maintaining connections with his friends and family. Each day brought new challenges and discoveries, but nothing could have prepared him for the unexpected revelations that were about to unfold.

One afternoon, as Alex was reviewing data in the lab, Dr. Vasquez approached him with a serious expression. "Alex, there's something we need to discuss. It's about the new compound we've been working on."

Concerned by her tone, Alex followed her to her office. Dr. Vasquez closed the door and handed him a stack of documents. "We've discovered some anomalies in the data. There are inconsistencies that suggest someone may have tampered with the results."

Alex's heart sank. "Tampered? But why would anyone do that?"

"We don't know yet," Dr. Vasquez replied, her voice filled with frustration. "But this could jeopardize all of our work. We need to find out who is responsible and ensure the integrity of our research."

Determined to get to the bottom of the issue, Alex and Dr. Vasquez began a thorough investigation. They combed through the data, cross-referencing every piece of information and scrutinizing every detail. It was a painstaking process, but they were determined to uncover the truth.

One evening, as Alex was working late in the lab, he received a call from Jessica. "Alex, I heard about the issues with the data. Is everything okay?"

Alex sighed, grateful for her concern. "It's been tough, Jess. We're still trying to figure out what happened. But I won't let this derail us."

"You've always been resilient, Alex," Jessica said, her voice filled with encouragement. "Just remember, you're not alone. We're all here for you."

The support of his friends was a constant source of strength for Alex. Emily, Sam, and Jessica checked in regularly, offering words of encouragement and helping him stay grounded. Their unwavering belief in him gave Alex the determination to keep pushing forward.

As the investigation progressed, Alex and Dr. Vasquez uncovered a trail of suspicious activity. The anomalies pointed to a new research assistant who had recently joined the team. Confronted with the evidence, the assistant confessed to altering the data in an attempt to accelerate their career.

The revelation was a shock to the entire team. Dr. Vasquez addressed the situation with firm resolve, ensuring that the assistant was removed from the project and the integrity of their research was restored. "We must remain vigilant and uphold the highest standards of our work," she said. "Our mission is too important to be compromised."

With the issue resolved, Alex and the team redoubled their efforts to validate their findings. The setback had been challenging, but it had also reinforced the importance of their work and the need for diligence and integrity.

One day, as Alex was reviewing the latest results, Dr. Vasquez approached him with a smile. "Alex, I have some good news. Despite the challenges we've faced, our latest tests confirm the efficacy of the new compound. This could be a significant breakthrough in treating Alzheimer's disease."

A wave of relief and excitement washed over Alex. "That's incredible, Dr. Vasquez. I'm so glad our hard work paid off."

"The journey has been difficult, but your dedication and perseverance have made all the difference," Dr. Vasquez said. "I believe this is just the beginning of what we can achieve."

As the news of their breakthrough spread, Alex found himself reflecting on the unexpected twists and turns of his journey. The challenges had tested his limits, but they had also revealed his resilience and capacity for growth.

Gathering with Emily, Sam, and Jessica to celebrate, Alex raised his glass in a toast. "To unexpected revelations and the strength to overcome them. We've faced many challenges, but we've also achieved so much. Here's to continuing this journey together."

"To resilience and friendship," Emily echoed, clinking her glass with his.

"And to the incredible journey ahead," Sam added.

Jessica smiled warmly. "We've come a long way, and I'm proud of us all. Here's to whatever comes next."

As they celebrated, Alex felt a profound sense of gratitude. The road ahead would undoubtedly hold more challenges, but with the support of his friends, mentors, and the knowledge that their work was making a tangible difference, he knew they could overcome anything together.

Chapter 19: The Final Push

The breakthrough in their research had reinvigorated the team at the International Institute for Neurological Research. The successful validation of the new compound marked a significant milestone, but Alex knew there was still much work to be done. As they entered the final phase of their project, the pressure intensified, and the stakes grew higher.

One morning, Alex received an email from Dr. Vasquez. "Alex, please come to my office as soon as possible. We need to discuss an urgent matter." Concerned by the urgency, Alex hurried to her office.

"Dr. Vasquez, what's going on?" Alex asked as he entered the room.

Dr. Vasquez looked up from her desk, her expression serious. "Alex, we've just received news that our project has been selected for accelerated clinical trials. This is a rare opportunity, but it also means we need to expedite our preparations."

Alex felt a surge of excitement and anxiety. "That's incredible news, but we have so much to do."

Dr. Vasquez nodded. "Indeed. We'll need to finalize our protocols, gather additional data, and ensure everything is in place for the trials. It's going to be an intense period, but I believe we can do it."

Determined to rise to the challenge, Alex and the team threw themselves into their work. The lab became a hive of activity as they conducted final tests, reviewed data, and prepared detailed reports for the clinical trials. The hours were long and the demands relentless, but the sense of purpose and urgency kept them going.

One evening, as Alex was working late in the lab, he received a call from Emily. "Hey, Alex. How's everything going with the project?"

"It's intense, Emily," Alex admitted, rubbing his tired eyes. "We're in the final push to get everything ready for the clinical trials. How are you?"

"We're all rooting for you, Alex," Emily said, her voice filled with support. "Just remember to take care of yourself. We can't wait to hear about your success."

The encouragement from his friends was a lifeline for Alex. He took short breaks to check in with Emily, Sam, and Jessica, their words of support providing much-needed motivation. Their unwavering belief in him fueled his determination to see the project through.

As the deadline approached, the pressure mounted. Alex and his colleagues worked around the clock, driven by the knowledge that their efforts could make a real difference in the lives of patients suffering from neurodegenerative diseases. The final days were a blur of activity, but the team's dedication and collaboration were unwavering.

On the eve of the deadline, Dr. Vasquez called a meeting. "I want to thank each of you for your incredible hard work and commitment," she said, her voice filled with pride. "We've accomplished something remarkable, and now it's time to submit our work and prepare for the clinical trials."

The team gathered in the conference room, reviewing the final documents and ensuring every detail was in order. As they submitted their work, a sense of relief and accomplishment washed over them. They had done everything in their power to prepare for the next phase.

The following weeks were a waiting game as they anticipated the start of the clinical trials. Alex took the opportunity to reconnect with his friends and family, finding solace in their company. The support of his loved ones had been instrumental in getting him this far, and he cherished the moments of respite.

One evening, as Alex was having dinner with Emily, Sam, and Jessica, his phone buzzed with an email notification. His heart raced as he saw it was from the clinical trial board. "It's from the board," he said, his voice trembling with anticipation.

"Open it, Alex!" Sam urged, his eyes wide with excitement.

Alex took a deep breath and opened the email. A broad smile spread across his face as he read the words. "We've been approved. The clinical trials are a go!"

The table erupted in cheers and applause. "That's amazing, Alex!" Emily exclaimed, hugging him tightly. "We knew you could do it."

Jessica raised her glass in a toast. "To Alex and the incredible work you've done. Here's to the clinical trials and the hope they bring."

"To Alex and the team," Sam added, clinking his glass with the others.

As they celebrated, Alex felt a profound sense of fulfillment. The journey had been long and challenging, but the approval for the clinical trials marked a significant achievement. With the support of his friends, mentors, and the dedication of his team, Alex felt ready to face the next chapter of their research.

As the clinical trials began, Alex and the team closely monitored the patients' progress. The initial results were promising, bringing a renewed sense of hope and purpose. The road ahead was still long, but the progress they had made was a testament to their resilience and determination.

One evening, as Alex reflected on the journey, he felt a deep sense of gratitude. The challenges, setbacks, and triumphs had shaped him in ways he never imagined. With the support of his friends, mentors, and the unwavering belief in their mission, he knew they could overcome any obstacle.

Gathering with his friends once more, Alex raised his glass in a toast. "To the final push and the incredible journey we've shared. Here's to the future and the endless possibilities it holds."

"To the future," Emily echoed, clinking her glass with his.

"And to the power of perseverance," Sam added.

Jessica smiled warmly. "We've come a long way, and I'm excited to see where the journey takes us next."

As they celebrated, Alex felt a profound sense of anticipation and readiness. The road ahead would undoubtedly hold more challenges, but with the strength of their bonds and the knowledge that their work was making a tangible difference, he knew they were ready to face whatever came next.

Chapter 20: Triumph and New Beginnings

The clinical trials marked a significant milestone in Alex's journey, but they were just the beginning. As the trials progressed, the team meticulously monitored the results, analyzing data, and making necessary adjustments. The initial success fueled their determination to push forward, but they knew the road ahead would still be challenging.

One morning, Alex received an unexpected call from Dr. Harris. "Alex, I have some exciting news. The preliminary results from the clinical trials are extremely promising. The patients are showing significant improvement, and the medical community is taking notice."

Alex felt a surge of excitement and relief. "That's incredible, Dr. Harris. I'm so glad our work is making a difference."

"This is just the beginning, Alex," Dr. Harris continued. "We've been invited to present our findings at the World Congress of Neurology. This is a huge platform, and it will give us the opportunity to share our breakthrough with the global medical community."

The prospect of presenting at such a prestigious conference was both exhilarating and daunting. Alex and Dr. Vasquez spent countless hours preparing their presentation, refining their data, and rehearsing their delivery. The support of their colleagues and the encouragement from their friends fueled their determination to make the most of this opportunity.

The day of the presentation arrived, and Alex felt a mix of nerves and excitement as he took the stage. The auditorium was filled with leading neurologists, researchers, and medical professionals from around the world. Alex began the presentation, highlighting the innovative approach they had taken and the promising results they had achieved.

As he spoke, Alex felt a surge of confidence. The audience listened intently, and when he concluded, the room erupted in applause. The positive reception was overwhelming, and Alex felt a deep sense of accomplishment.

After the presentation, Alex was approached by several prominent figures in the field. "Your work is truly groundbreaking," one of them said. "We'd like to discuss potential collaborations and further research opportunities."

The recognition and interest from the global medical community opened new doors for Alex and his team. They returned to the institute with renewed energy and a clear vision for the future. The next phase of their research would involve expanding the clinical trials, exploring new treatment protocols, and continuing to push the boundaries of what was possible.

As the months passed, the impact of their work became increasingly evident. The patients in the clinical trials continued to show improvement, and the positive results were published in leading medical journals. The success of the project brought a sense of fulfillment and pride to everyone involved.

One evening, as Alex was reflecting on the journey, he received a call from his father. "Alex, I have some wonderful news. Your mother's latest tests show remarkable improvement. The doctors are optimistic about her recovery."

Tears of joy filled Alex's eyes. "That's amazing, Dad. I'm so happy to hear it."

The progress his mother had made was a testament to the importance of their work and the real impact it had on patients' lives. It reinforced Alex's commitment to continue pushing forward, driven by the knowledge that their research was making a tangible difference.

As the year drew to a close, the institute held a celebration to honor the achievements of the team. Colleagues, friends, and family gathered to celebrate the milestones they had reached and the promise of the future. Dr. Vasquez took the stage to address the crowd.

"I want to extend my heartfelt gratitude to each and every one of you for your dedication and hard work," she said. "This year has been filled with challenges, but also with triumphs. Our success is a testament to the power of collaboration, perseverance, and the unwavering belief in our mission."

Alex felt a surge of pride as Dr. Vasquez continued. "I especially want to acknowledge Alex for his remarkable contributions. His leadership, innovation, and dedication have been instrumental in our success. We are incredibly proud of what we've achieved together and excited for the future."

As the celebration continued, Alex raised his glass in a toast. "To triumphs and new beginnings. We've faced many challenges, but we've also accomplished so much. Here's to the incredible journey ahead and the endless possibilities it holds."

"To the future," Emily echoed, clinking her glass with his.

"And to the strength of our bonds," Sam added.

Jessica smiled warmly. "We've come a long way, and I'm proud of us all. Here's to whatever comes next."

As they celebrated, Alex felt a profound sense of gratitude and anticipation. The journey had been transformative, shaping him into the person he was today. With the support of his friends, mentors, and the knowledge that their work was making a difference, Alex felt ready to embrace the future with confidence and determination.

Chapter 21: Reflections and Future Paths

The achievements of the past year had set a new benchmark for Alex and his team at the International Institute for Neurological Research. As the initial phase of the clinical trials concluded, the positive results reinforced their commitment to pushing the boundaries of medical science. However, with these successes came the need for reflection and planning for the future.

One crisp winter morning, Alex received a call from Dr. Matthews. "Alex, I've been following your progress closely, and I'm incredibly proud of what you've accomplished. I think it's time for us to discuss the next steps in your career."

Excited by the prospect, Alex scheduled a meeting with Dr. Matthews. They met in Dr. Matthews' office, a place that held many memories of Alex's early days at MedTech University.

"Alex, your work has been outstanding," Dr. Matthews began, a proud smile on his face. "You've made significant contributions to the field of neurology, and I believe you're ready for a new challenge."

Alex leaned forward, eager to hear more. "What do you have in mind, Dr. Matthews?"

"I've been in discussions with several institutions about forming a collaborative research initiative focused on neurodegenerative diseases," Dr. Matthews explained. "We want you to lead this initiative. It will be a multidisciplinary team bringing together experts from around the world."

The proposal was both exhilarating and daunting. Alex felt a mix of excitement and responsibility. "I'm honored, Dr. Matthews. This is an incredible opportunity. I'd love to be part of it."

"Excellent," Dr. Matthews said, his eyes twinkling with enthusiasm. "I have no doubt that you'll lead this initiative with the same dedication and passion you've shown throughout your career."

With the support of Dr. Matthews and his colleagues, Alex began to lay the groundwork for the new research initiative. He reached out to leading experts in various fields, coordinating meetings and building a team that shared his vision. The collaborative nature of the initiative brought together diverse perspectives, fostering an environment of innovation and creativity.

As Alex navigated the complexities of establishing the new initiative, he found himself reflecting on his journey. The challenges, setbacks, and triumphs had shaped him into the leader he was today. He took time to reconnect with his friends, whose unwavering support had been a cornerstone of his success.

One evening, Alex hosted a dinner to celebrate the launch of the research initiative. Emily, Sam, and Jessica joined him, their camaraderie and laughter filling the room with warmth.

"To new beginnings," Alex said, raising his glass. "We've come a long way, and I couldn't have done it without all of you. Here's to the incredible journey ahead."

"To new beginnings," Emily echoed, clinking her glass with his.

"And to the strength of our friendships," Sam added.

Jessica smiled warmly. "We've faced so much together, and I'm excited to see where this journey takes us next."

As they celebrated, Alex felt a profound sense of gratitude. The journey had been transformative, not just for him, but for everyone who had been part of it. The new research initiative represented not just a professional milestone, but a testament to the power of collaboration, resilience, and the unwavering belief in their mission.

In the weeks that followed, Alex threw himself into the work of the new initiative. The collaborative team began to explore new avenues of research, pushing the boundaries of what was possible. The challenges were significant, but the potential impact of their work drove them forward.

One afternoon, as Alex was reviewing data in his office, he received a call from Dr. Vasquez. "Alex, I wanted to congratulate you on the launch of the new initiative. Your leadership and vision are truly inspiring."

"Thank you, Dr. Vasquez," Alex replied, feeling a deep sense of pride. "I'm excited about the possibilities ahead. Our work has the potential to make a real difference."

"And it will," Dr. Vasquez affirmed. "You've already shown what's possible with dedication and innovation. I'm confident that this initiative will achieve great things."

As Alex hung up the phone, he felt a renewed sense of purpose. The journey ahead would undoubtedly hold more challenges, but with the support of his friends, mentors, and colleagues, he knew they were ready to face whatever came next.

Gathering his team for a meeting, Alex looked around at the faces of the brilliant minds he had brought together. "We have an incredible opportunity to push the boundaries of medical science and make a real difference in the lives of patients. Let's work together, support each other, and achieve something truly remarkable."

The team responded with enthusiasm, their collective energy and dedication palpable. As they began their work, Alex felt a profound sense of fulfillment. The journey had been long and challenging, but it had also been incredibly rewarding.

With the strength of their bonds and the knowledge that their work was making a tangible difference, Alex and his team were ready to embrace the future with confidence and determination. The horizon was filled with endless possibilities, and they were eager to explore them, one breakthrough at a time.

Chapter 22: Challenges Ahead

The launch of the new research initiative brought a renewed sense of purpose and excitement to Alex and his team. The collaborative effort had already begun to yield promising results, but they knew that significant challenges lay ahead. The path to groundbreaking discoveries was fraught with obstacles, and it would take resilience, innovation, and unwavering determination to overcome them.

One morning, as Alex was reviewing the latest data, he received an urgent call from Dr. Matthews. "Alex, there's been a development that requires your immediate attention. Can you come to my office?"

Concerned by the urgency in Dr. Matthews' voice, Alex quickly made his way to the office. He found Dr. Matthews deep in conversation with Dr. Vasquez, both looking unusually serious.

"What's going on?" Alex asked, feeling a knot of anxiety form in his stomach.

Dr. Matthews gestured for him to sit. "We've encountered a significant setback in our trials. Some patients have developed unexpected complications, and we need to investigate the cause immediately."

Alex felt a surge of concern. The success of their initiative hinged on the safety and efficacy of their treatments. "What kind of complications are we seeing?"

Dr. Vasquez sighed. "Some patients are experiencing severe adverse reactions that we hadn't anticipated. We need to halt the trials temporarily and conduct a thorough investigation."

The news was a blow to the team, but Alex knew they couldn't afford to lose momentum. "Let's get to work. We need to identify the cause and find a solution as quickly as possible."

The following weeks were a whirlwind of activity as the team delved into the data, analyzing every detail to uncover the source of the complications. The pressure was immense, but the stakes were too high to falter. Alex and his colleagues worked around the clock, driven by a shared commitment to their mission.

One evening, as Alex was poring over data in the lab, Emily called to check in. "Hey, Alex. I heard about the complications. How are you holding up?"

"It's been tough, Emily," Alex admitted, rubbing his tired eyes. "But we can't give up. These patients are counting on us."

"You're doing incredible work, Alex," Emily said, her voice filled with encouragement. "Just remember, you're not alone. We're all here to support you."

The support of his friends was a lifeline for Alex. Emily, Sam, and Jessica kept in regular contact, offering words of encouragement and helping him stay grounded. Their unwavering belief in him fueled his determination to keep pushing forward.

As the investigation progressed, the team made a breakthrough. They identified a specific genetic marker that was linked to the adverse reactions, allowing them to refine the treatment protocol and mitigate the risks. The discovery brought a wave of relief and renewed hope.

Dr. Vasquez called a meeting to announce the findings. "Thanks to our team's hard work, we've identified the cause of the complications and implemented a solution. This is a significant step forward, and I want to commend Alex for his exceptional contributions."

The room erupted in applause, and Alex felt a surge of pride and gratitude. The journey had been challenging, but the outcome was worth every effort.

As the trials resumed, the team closely monitored the patients' progress, making adjustments as needed. The initial results were promising, bringing a renewed sense of optimism and purpose. The road ahead was still long, but the progress they had made was a testament to their resilience and dedication.

One evening, as Alex was reflecting on the journey, he received a call from his father. "Alex, I have some good news. Your mother's latest tests show continued improvement. The doctors are very pleased with her progress."

Tears of relief filled Alex's eyes. "That's wonderful, Dad. I'm so glad to hear it."

The progress his mother had made was a constant reminder of the importance of their work and the real impact it had on patients' lives. It reinforced Alex's commitment to continue pushing forward, driven by the knowledge that their research was making a tangible difference.

Gathering with his friends to celebrate, Alex raised his glass in a toast. "To resilience and the strength to overcome challenges. We've faced many obstacles, but we've also achieved so much. Here's to the incredible journey ahead and the endless possibilities it holds."

"To resilience and friendship," Emily echoed, clinking her glass with his.

"And to the power of perseverance," Sam added.

Jessica smiled warmly. "We've come a long way, and I'm excited to see where the journey takes us next."

As they celebrated, Alex felt a profound sense of gratitude and anticipation. The journey had been transformative, shaping him into the person he was today. With the support of his friends, mentors, and the unwavering belief in their mission, he knew they were ready to face whatever challenges lay ahead.

Chapter 23: Breaking Barriers

The research initiative had reached a critical juncture. With the trials back on track and initial results looking promising, Alex and his team knew they were on the verge of something groundbreaking. The sense of anticipation was palpable, and the team worked with renewed vigor, determined to break through the remaining barriers.

One morning, Alex received an email from a leading pharmaceutical company interested in their research. "We are impressed with your preliminary findings and would like to discuss potential collaboration and funding opportunities," the email read.

Excited by the prospect, Alex shared the news with Dr. Vasquez. "This could be a game-changer for our project," he said. "With additional funding and resources, we could accelerate our progress and reach more patients."

Dr. Vasquez nodded, her eyes gleaming with enthusiasm. "Let's set up a meeting and explore this opportunity further."

The following week, Alex and Dr. Vasquez met with representatives from the pharmaceutical company. The discussions were productive, and the company expressed strong interest in supporting their research. The potential collaboration promised not only financial backing but also access to cutting-edge technology and a broader platform to share their findings.

As the team finalized the partnership, Alex reflected on the journey that had brought them to this point. The challenges they had faced had only strengthened their resolve, and the support from the pharmaceutical company was a testament to the impact of their work.

With the new partnership in place, the team expanded their research efforts. They hired additional staff, acquired advanced equipment, and initiated more extensive clinical trials. The pace was intense, but the sense of purpose and the potential to make a significant difference drove them forward.

One evening, as Alex was reviewing data in the lab, he received a call from Emily. "Hey, Alex. How are things going with the new partnership?"

"It's been incredible, Emily," Alex replied, a note of excitement in his voice. "The support from the pharmaceutical company has really boosted our efforts. We're making great progress."

"I'm so happy for you, Alex," Emily said, her voice filled with pride. "You've worked so hard for this, and it's paying off."

The encouragement from his friends continued to be a source of strength for Alex. Emily, Sam, and Jessica remained steadfast in their support, offering words of encouragement and celebrating each milestone with him.

As the months passed, the team made significant strides in their research. The expanded clinical trials yielded positive results, and the data showed that their treatment could not only slow the progression of neurodegenerative diseases but also improve patients' quality of life.

The success of their work attracted attention from the global medical community. Alex was invited to speak at several international conferences, where he shared their findings and collaborated with other leading researchers. The recognition and validation from his peers were both humbling and motivating.

One day, as Alex was preparing for a presentation at a major medical conference, he received a call from Dr. Harris. "Alex, I wanted to personally congratulate you on the incredible progress you've made. Your work is truly groundbreaking."

"Thank you, Dr. Harris," Alex replied, feeling a deep sense of gratitude. "Your guidance and support have been invaluable throughout this journey."

"Keep pushing forward, Alex," Dr. Harris said. "The work you're doing is making a real difference, and I have no doubt that you'll continue to achieve great things."

The conference was a resounding success, and Alex's presentation received widespread acclaim. The positive feedback and interest from the global medical community reinforced the importance of their work and the potential for future breakthroughs.

As the team returned to the institute, they were greeted with news that their research had been nominated for a prestigious medical award. The nomination was a testament to their hard work and dedication, and it brought a sense of pride and accomplishment to everyone involved.

Gathering with his friends to celebrate, Alex raised his glass in a toast. "To breaking barriers and the incredible journey we've shared. We've faced many challenges, but we've also achieved so much. Here's to the future and the endless possibilities it holds."

"To breaking barriers," Emily echoed, clinking her glass with his.

"And to the power of perseverance," Sam added.

Jessica smiled warmly. "We've come a long way, and I'm excited to see where the journey takes us next."

As they celebrated, Alex felt a profound sense of gratitude and anticipation. The journey had been transformative, shaping him into the leader he was today. With the support of his friends, mentors, and the unwavering belief in their mission, he knew they were ready to face whatever challenges lay ahead.

Chapter 24: The Pinnacle of Achievement

The recognition and accolades had brought a sense of accomplishment to Alex and his team, but they knew their journey was far from over. The work they had done was a significant step forward, but there were still many questions to answer and many patients to help. The team's commitment to pushing the boundaries of medical science remained unwavering.

One morning, as Alex was preparing for another day in the lab, he received an email from the Nobel Committee. The subject line read, "Nomination for the Nobel Prize in Medicine." His heart raced as he opened the email, scarcely believing what he was seeing.

"Dear Dr. Alexander Carter,

We are pleased to inform you that you and your team have been nominated for the Nobel Prize in Medicine for your groundbreaking work in the treatment of neurodegenerative diseases. Your innovative research has made significant contributions to the field, and we look forward to discussing your achievements further.

Congratulations on this prestigious nomination.

Best regards,
The Nobel Committee"

Alex felt a wave of disbelief and excitement. He quickly shared the news with Dr. Vasquez and the rest of the team, who responded with cheers and applause.

"This is an incredible honor," Dr. Vasquez said, her eyes shining with pride. "It's a testament to the hard work and dedication of everyone involved."

As the news spread, the excitement grew. The nomination brought with it a whirlwind of media attention, interviews, and preparations for the Nobel Prize ceremony. Alex and his team were invited to present their work at several high-profile events, further solidifying their reputation as leaders in the field.

In the weeks leading up to the ceremony, Alex reflected on the journey that had brought them to this point. The challenges, setbacks, and triumphs had shaped them into a resilient and determined team. The support of his friends, mentors, and colleagues had been instrumental in their success.

One evening, as Alex was preparing for an upcoming presentation, he received a call from his father. "Alex, your mother and I are so proud of you. Your nomination for the Nobel Prize is an incredible achievement."

"Thanks, Dad," Alex replied, his voice filled with emotion. "I couldn't have done it without your support."

"We always believed in you, Alex," his father said. "Your work is making a real difference, and that's something to be incredibly proud of."

As the day of the Nobel Prize ceremony approached, the anticipation and excitement reached new heights. The ceremony was held in Stockholm, and Alex felt a mix of nerves and pride as he prepared to take the stage. He was surrounded by the world's leading scientists, researchers, and dignitaries, all gathered to celebrate the achievements in medicine.

When Alex's name was called, he took a deep breath and walked to the stage. The applause was deafening, and he felt a profound sense of gratitude as he accepted the Nobel Prize in Medicine on behalf of his team.

"Thank you," Alex began, his voice steady. "This award is a testament to the incredible work of my team and the unwavering support of our friends and families. Our journey has been filled with challenges, but it has also been incredibly rewarding. We are committed to continuing our work and pushing the boundaries of medical science to improve the lives of patients around the world."

As he left the stage, Alex felt a deep sense of fulfillment. The recognition was a significant milestone, but it was also a reminder of the importance of their work and the impact it could have.

In the days following the ceremony, Alex and his team were inundated with congratulations and offers of collaboration from leading institutions and researchers. The Nobel Prize had opened new doors and provided a platform to further their research and reach even more patients.

Gathering with his friends to celebrate, Alex raised his glass in a toast. "To the pinnacle of achievement and the incredible journey we've shared. We've faced many challenges, but we've also accomplished so much. Here's to the future and the endless possibilities it holds."

"To the future," Emily echoed, clinking her glass with his.

"And to the power of perseverance," Sam added.

Jessica smiled warmly. "We've come a long way, and I'm excited to see where the journey takes us next."

As they celebrated, Alex felt a profound sense of gratitude and anticipation. The journey had been transformative, shaping him into the leader he was today. With the support of his friends, mentors, and the unwavering belief in their mission, he knew they were ready to face whatever challenges lay ahead.

Chapter 25: The Legacy Continues

The Nobel Prize ceremony had been a pinnacle moment for Alex and his team, but it also marked the beginning of a new chapter in their journey. The recognition and accolades had brought new opportunities, and the team was more determined than ever to push the boundaries of medical science and improve the lives of patients worldwide.

One morning, as Alex was reflecting on the recent events, he received a call from Dr. Vasquez. "Alex, I've been thinking about the future of our research and the impact we want to have. I believe it's time for us to expand our efforts and establish a global research network."

Intrigued by the idea, Alex met with Dr. Vasquez to discuss the details. "A global research network would allow us to collaborate with leading experts from around the world, share knowledge, and accelerate our progress," Dr. Vasquez explained. "I believe you are the right person to lead this initiative."

Alex felt a mix of excitement and responsibility. "Thank you, Dr. Vasquez. I am honored by your trust. Let's build something truly remarkable."

With the support of the institute and the pharmaceutical company, Alex began laying the groundwork for the global research network. He reached out to leading institutions and researchers, coordinating meetings and building partnerships. The response was overwhelmingly positive, and the network quickly began to take shape.

The launch of the Global Neurological Research Network (GNRN) was a significant milestone. The collaborative effort brought together brilliant minds from various disciplines, fostering an environment of innovation and creativity. The GNRN aimed to address some of the most pressing challenges in neurology, from neurodegenerative diseases to brain injuries and beyond.

As the network expanded, Alex and his team worked tirelessly to coordinate research efforts, share data, and develop new treatment protocols. The collaborative approach accelerated their progress, leading to several breakthroughs in a short period.

One evening, as Alex was working late in his office, he received a call from Emily. "Hey, Alex. How's everything going with the GNRN?"

"It's been incredible, Emily," Alex replied, his voice filled with enthusiasm. "The collaboration and support from researchers worldwide have been amazing. We're making real progress."

"I'm so proud of you, Alex," Emily said, her voice filled with admiration. "You've come a long way, and you're making a real difference."

The encouragement from his friends continued to be a source of strength for Alex. Emily, Sam, and Jessica remained steadfast in their support, celebrating each milestone and offering words of encouragement.

As the GNRN grew, the team published several groundbreaking studies that garnered international attention. Their work was featured in leading medical journals, and Alex was invited to speak at numerous conferences. The recognition reinforced the importance of their mission and the impact of their collaborative efforts.

One day, while reviewing the latest research findings, Alex received an email from a prestigious university offering him a professorship. The opportunity to teach and mentor the next generation of researchers was an exciting prospect.

After discussing the offer with Dr. Vasquez, Alex decided to accept the position. "I believe this will allow me to continue our work while also inspiring and guiding young researchers," he explained.

The transition to academia was a new challenge, but Alex embraced it with the same dedication and passion that had driven his research. He established a research lab at the university, continuing his work with the GNRN while also teaching and mentoring students.

One evening, as Alex was preparing for a lecture, he received a call from his father. "Alex, I wanted to tell you how proud we are of you. Your mother and I have been following your work, and it's truly inspiring."

"Thanks, Dad," Alex replied, his voice filled with emotion. "Your support has meant everything to me."

As Alex stood in front of his class the next day, he felt a profound sense of fulfillment. The journey had been long and challenging, but it had also been incredibly rewarding. He was surrounded by bright young minds eager to learn and make a difference.

In his lecture, Alex shared his experiences, emphasizing the importance of resilience, collaboration, and the unwavering belief in their mission. "Our work is far from over," he said. "But together, we can continue to push the boundaries of medical science and improve the lives of patients worldwide."

The students listened intently, their eyes filled with admiration and hope. Alex felt a deep sense of pride, knowing that the legacy of their work would continue through the next generation of researchers.

As the semester progressed, Alex balanced his responsibilities at the university with his ongoing work with the GNRN. The network continued to thrive, producing groundbreaking research and fostering international collaboration.

Gathering with his friends to celebrate another successful year, Alex raised his glass in a toast. "To the legacy we are building and the incredible journey we've shared. We've faced many challenges, but we've also achieved so much. Here's to the future and the endless possibilities it holds."

"To the legacy," Emily echoed, clinking her glass with his.

"And to the power of perseverance," Sam added.

Jessica smiled warmly. "We've come a long way, and I'm excited to see where the journey takes us next."

As they celebrated, Alex felt a profound sense of gratitude and anticipation. The journey had been transformative, shaping him into the leader he was today. With the support of his friends, mentors, and the unwavering belief in their mission, he knew they were ready to face whatever challenges lay ahead.

Chapter 26: Embracing the Future

With the establishment of the Global Neurological Research Network (GNRN) and his new role in academia, Alex's life had reached a fulfilling yet demanding balance. The journey thus far had been filled with triumphs and challenges, shaping him into a leader and mentor. However, he knew that the future held even more opportunities and obstacles to navigate.

One morning, as Alex was preparing for a lecture, he received an email from an unexpected source: the World Health Organization (WHO). The subject line read, "Invitation to Join the Global Health Advisory Board." Intrigued, Alex quickly opened the email.

"Dear Dr. Alexander Carter,

We are pleased to extend an invitation for you to join the Global Health Advisory Board. Your groundbreaking work in neurology and your leadership in the Global Neurological Research Network have made significant impacts on global health. We believe your expertise and insights will be invaluable in shaping health policies and advancing medical research on an international scale.

We look forward to your positive response.

Best regards,
Dr. Margaret Hinton
Director-General, World Health Organization"

Alex felt a surge of excitement and pride. The opportunity to influence global health policies and contribute to medical research at an international level was a dream come true. He immediately shared the news with Dr. Vasquez and his team.

"This is an incredible honor, Alex," Dr. Vasquez said, her eyes shining with pride. "Your work is truly making a global impact."

With the support of his colleagues and friends, Alex accepted the invitation. The new role brought additional responsibilities, including international travel, policy discussions, and collaborations with global health leaders. Balancing his commitments at the university, the GNRN, and the WHO was challenging, but Alex thrived on the dynamic environment and the potential to make a broader impact.

One evening, as Alex was preparing for a conference call with the WHO, he received a call from Emily. "Hey, Alex. How's everything going with your new role?"

"It's been intense, Emily," Alex admitted, "but incredibly rewarding. The opportunity to influence global health policies is amazing."

"We're all so proud of you, Alex," Emily said, her voice filled with admiration. "You've come so far, and you're making a real difference."

The support from his friends continued to be a source of strength for Alex. Emily, Sam, and Jessica remained steadfast in their encouragement, celebrating each milestone and offering words of wisdom.

As the months passed, Alex's influence in the global health community grew. He played a key role in shaping policies and initiatives aimed at addressing neurological diseases and improving healthcare access worldwide. His work with the WHO, combined with his ongoing research and teaching, positioned him as a leading figure in the field of neurology.

One day, while attending a global health summit, Alex was approached by Dr. Margaret Hinton. "Alex, your contributions to our initiatives have been invaluable. Your insights and dedication are truly inspiring."

"Thank you, Dr. Hinton," Alex replied, feeling a deep sense of pride. "It's an honor to be part of this important work."

As the summit continued, Alex engaged in discussions with health leaders from around the world, sharing knowledge and forging new partnerships. The collaborative spirit and shared commitment to improving global health reinforced his belief in the power of teamwork and perseverance.

Returning to the university, Alex found himself reflecting on the journey that had brought him to this point. The challenges, setbacks, and triumphs had shaped him into a leader with a vision for the future. He was surrounded by brilliant minds, eager students, and supportive friends and colleagues, all working towards a common goal.

Gathering with his friends to celebrate another successful year, Alex raised his glass in a toast. "To embracing the future and the incredible journey we've shared. We've faced many challenges, but we've also achieved so much. Here's to the endless possibilities that lie ahead."

"To the future," Emily echoed, clinking her glass with his.

"And to the power of perseverance," Sam added.

Jessica smiled warmly. "We've come a long way, and I'm excited to see where the journey takes us next."

As they celebrated, Alex felt a profound sense of gratitude and anticipation. The journey had been transformative, shaping him into the leader he was today. With the support of his friends, mentors, and the unwavering belief in their mission, he knew they were ready to face whatever challenges lay ahead.

As the evening drew to a close, Alex stood on the balcony, looking out over the city. The future was filled with uncertainty, but also with boundless potential. Embracing the future meant continuing to push the boundaries of medical science, inspiring the next generation of researchers, and making a lasting impact on global health.

With a sense of determination and hope, Alex turned back to join his friends, ready to embrace whatever the future held.

Chapter 27: The Uncharted Path

With each passing day, the Global Neurological Research Network (GNRN) and Alex's influence in the field of neurology continued to grow. The success and recognition were rewarding, but Alex knew that the path forward would be filled with new challenges and uncharted territories. The commitment to pushing the boundaries of medical science and improving global health required constant innovation and resilience.

One afternoon, as Alex was reviewing a new research proposal, he received a call from Dr. Matthews. "Alex, I need to discuss an urgent matter with you. Can you come to my office?"

Concerned by the tone of his voice, Alex made his way to Dr. Matthews' office. He found his mentor deep in thought, surrounded by documents and data.

"What's going on, Dr. Matthews?" Alex asked, taking a seat.

Dr. Matthews looked up, his expression serious. "Alex, we've encountered a potential breakthrough in our research, but it involves uncharted territory. The data suggests a novel approach to treating neurodegenerative diseases, but it comes with significant risks."

Alex felt a surge of curiosity and determination. "What kind of risks are we talking about?"

Dr. Matthews handed him a stack of documents. "The new approach involves gene editing and targeted therapies. While the preliminary results are promising, the long-term effects and potential side effects are still unknown. We need to proceed with caution and rigor."

Alex nodded, absorbing the information. "I understand the risks, but this could be a game-changer for our patients. Let's gather the team and discuss the best way forward."

Over the next few days, Alex and his team delved into the new approach, analyzing data, conducting experiments, and weighing the potential benefits and risks. The discussions were intense, with varying opinions on how to proceed. Some team members were excited by the potential breakthrough, while others were concerned about the ethical implications and safety.

One evening, as Alex was deep in thought, Emily called to check in. "Hey, Alex. How are things going with the new research?"

"It's been challenging, Emily," Alex admitted. "We're exploring uncharted territory, and the stakes are high. But I believe this could make a significant difference for our patients."

"You've always been willing to take on challenges, Alex," Emily said, her voice filled with encouragement. "Just remember, you're not alone. We're all here to support you."

The support from his friends continued to be a source of strength for Alex. Emily, Sam, and Jessica remained steadfast in their encouragement, offering words of wisdom and helping him stay grounded.

As the team continued their work, they developed a comprehensive plan to test the new approach while minimizing risks. They decided to conduct a series of controlled trials, closely monitoring the patients and adjusting the treatment protocols as needed.

The initial trials were met with both successes and setbacks. Some patients showed remarkable improvement, while others experienced unexpected complications. The team worked tirelessly to refine their approach, learning from each trial and making necessary adjustments.

One day, while reviewing the latest trial results, Dr. Vasquez approached Alex with a thoughtful expression. "Alex, I want to commend you on your leadership and dedication. This journey has been filled with uncertainties, but your commitment to our mission has been unwavering."

"Thank you, Dr. Vasquez," Alex replied, feeling a deep sense of gratitude. "This work is important, and I'm grateful for the support of our incredible team."

As the months passed, the trials continued, and the team made significant progress. The refined approach showed promising results, with more patients experiencing positive outcomes. The data was encouraging, and the team felt a renewed sense of hope and purpose.

One evening, as Alex was reflecting on the journey, he received a call from his mother. "Alex, I wanted to tell you how proud I am of you. Your work is making a real difference, and I couldn't be prouder."

Tears of gratitude filled Alex's eyes. "Thank you, Mom. Your support means everything to me."

As the trials progressed, the team's work attracted attention from the global medical community. Alex was invited to present their findings at several international conferences, where he shared their innovative approach and the promising results.

Gathering with his friends to celebrate another milestone, Alex raised his glass in a toast. "To the uncharted path and the incredible journey we've shared. We've faced many challenges, but we've also achieved so much. Here's to the future and the endless possibilities it holds."

"To the uncharted path," Emily echoed, clinking her glass with his.

"And to the power of perseverance," Sam added.

Jessica smiled warmly. "We've come a long way, and I'm excited to see where the journey takes us next."

As they celebrated, Alex felt a profound sense of gratitude and anticipation. The journey had been transformative, shaping him into the leader he was today. With the support of his friends, mentors, and the unwavering belief in their mission, he knew they were ready to face whatever challenges lay ahead.

As the evening drew to a close, Alex stood on the balcony, looking out over the city. The future was filled with uncertainty, but also with boundless potential. Embracing the uncharted path meant continuing to push the boundaries of medical science, inspiring the next generation of researchers, and making a lasting impact on global health.

With a sense of determination and hope, Alex turned back to join his friends, ready to embrace whatever the future held.

Chapter 28: Resolute Determination

The trials had shown promising results, and Alex's team was on the cusp of a major breakthrough in treating neurodegenerative diseases. The sense of progress and purpose was palpable, but so were the challenges. The journey had been arduous, filled with moments of doubt and perseverance. Yet, Alex's determination remained unshaken.

One morning, as Alex was finalizing a report on the latest trial results, he received a call from Dr. Harris. "Alex, I've been reviewing your recent findings. The progress you've made is remarkable, but I believe there's still room for improvement. I think it's time we consider incorporating advanced AI algorithms to refine our data analysis."

Intrigued by the suggestion, Alex arranged a meeting with Dr. Harris and the AI research team. "Incorporating AI could enhance our ability to identify patterns and predict outcomes, but we'll need to ensure the algorithms are meticulously validated," Alex said.

The collaboration with the AI research team brought a new dimension to their work. The integration of machine learning algorithms enabled the team to process vast amounts of data with unprecedented accuracy. The insights gained from the AI analysis led to more precise treatment protocols and improved patient outcomes.

One evening, as Alex was reviewing the AI-generated data, he received a call from Emily. "Hey, Alex. How's everything going with the new AI integration?"

"It's been incredible, Emily," Alex replied, a note of excitement in his voice. "The AI algorithms have provided us with deeper insights and have already led to significant improvements in our treatment protocols."

"I'm so happy for you, Alex," Emily said, her voice filled with pride. "You've always been at the forefront of innovation."

The support from his friends continued to be a source of strength for

Alex. Emily, Sam, and Jessica remained steadfast in their encouragement, celebrating each milestone and offering words of wisdom.

As the months passed, the team's work attracted attention from the global medical community. Their innovative approach was published in leading medical journals, and Alex was invited to speak at several high-profile conferences. The recognition and validation from his peers reinforced the importance of their mission and the impact of their collaborative efforts.

One day, while preparing for a presentation at an international medical conference, Alex received a call from his father. "Alex, your mother and I have been following your work closely. We couldn't be prouder of all that you've accomplished."

"Thanks, Dad," Alex replied, his voice filled with emotion. "Your support has meant everything to me."

The conference was a resounding success, and Alex's presentation received widespread acclaim. The positive feedback and interest from the global medical community reinforced the importance of their work and the potential for future breakthroughs.

As the team returned to the institute, they were greeted with news that their research had been nominated for several prestigious awards. The nominations were a testament to their hard work and dedication, bringing a sense of pride and accomplishment to everyone involved.

Gathering with his friends to celebrate another milestone, Alex raised his glass in a toast. "To resolute determination and the incredible journey we've shared. We've faced many challenges, but we've also achieved so much. Here's to the future and the endless possibilities it holds."

"To determination and perseverance," Emily echoed, clinking her glass with his.

"And to the power of innovation," Sam added.

Jessica smiled warmly. "We've come a long way, and I'm excited to see where the journey takes us next."

As they celebrated, Alex felt a profound sense of gratitude and anticipation. The journey had been transformative, shaping him into the leader he was today. With the support of his friends, mentors, and the unwavering belief in their mission, he knew they were ready to face whatever challenges lay ahead.

One evening, as Alex stood on the balcony, looking out over the city, he felt a deep sense of fulfillment. The future was filled with uncertainty, but also with boundless potential. Embracing the future meant continuing to push the boundaries of medical science, inspiring the next generation of researchers, and making a lasting impact on global health.

With a sense of determination and hope, Alex turned back to join his friends, ready to embrace whatever the future held.

Chapter 29: A Vision for Tomorrow

As Alex and his team continued to push the boundaries of medical research, their efforts were beginning to shape a new future for neurological treatments. The integration of advanced AI algorithms had revolutionized their approach, allowing for unprecedented precision and effectiveness. The journey thus far had been filled with triumphs, challenges, and unyielding determination. Now, they stood at the threshold of new possibilities, ready to embrace the future with a clear vision.

One afternoon, Alex received an email from a prominent research institution in Europe. The subject line read, "Invitation to Collaborate on a Global Initiative." Intrigued, Alex opened the email and read the details of the proposed collaboration.

"Dear Dr. Alexander Carter,

We have been closely following your groundbreaking work in neurology and are impressed by your innovative approaches and significant contributions to the field. We would like to invite you to collaborate on a global initiative aimed at addressing neurological health disparities across different regions. Your expertise and leadership would be invaluable in shaping this initiative and driving its success.

We look forward to your positive response.

Best regards,
Dr. Elise Laurent
Director, European Institute of Neurological Research"

Excited by the opportunity, Alex immediately shared the news with Dr. Vasquez and the team. "This could be a transformative project, allowing us to extend our impact globally and address critical health disparities," Alex said.

Dr. Vasquez nodded in agreement. "It's an incredible opportunity, Alex.

Let's discuss the details and see how we can integrate our efforts."

Over the next few weeks, Alex and Dr. Vasquez worked closely with Dr. Laurent and her team to outline the objectives and strategies for the global initiative. The collaboration brought together leading experts from various regions, creating a diverse and dynamic team focused on addressing neurological health disparities.

One evening, as Alex was preparing for a video conference with the European team, he received a call from Emily. "Hey, Alex. How are things going with the new global initiative?"

"It's been incredibly rewarding, Emily," Alex replied, his voice filled with enthusiasm. "The collaboration and shared vision are inspiring. We're making real progress in addressing health disparities."

"I'm so proud of you, Alex," Emily said, her voice filled with admiration. "Your work is making a global impact."

The support from his friends continued to be a source of strength for Alex. Emily, Sam, and Jessica remained steadfast in their encouragement, celebrating each milestone and offering words of wisdom.

As the global initiative took shape, the team conducted extensive research, analyzed data from different regions, and developed targeted strategies to address the unique challenges faced by various communities. The collaborative effort led to several innovative solutions, improving access to neurological care and treatment outcomes.

One day, while attending a global health summit, Alex was approached by Dr. Laurent. "Alex, your leadership and vision have been instrumental in the success of this initiative. Your ability to bring together diverse perspectives and drive meaningful change is truly remarkable."

"Thank you, Dr. Laurent," Alex replied, feeling a deep sense of pride. "It's been an honor to work with such a dedicated and talented team."

As the summit continued, Alex engaged in discussions with health leaders from around the world, sharing knowledge and forging new partnerships. The collaborative spirit and shared commitment to improving global health reinforced his belief in the power of teamwork and perseverance.

Returning to the university, Alex found himself reflecting on the journey that had brought him to this point. The challenges, setbacks, and triumphs had shaped him into a leader with a vision for the future. He was surrounded by brilliant minds, eager students, and supportive friends and colleagues, all working towards a common goal.

Gathering with his friends to celebrate another successful year, Alex raised his glass in a toast. "To a vision for tomorrow and the incredible journey we've shared. We've faced many challenges, but we've also achieved so much. Here's to the future and the endless possibilities it holds."

"To the future," Emily echoed, clinking her glass with his.

"And to the power of perseverance," Sam added.

Jessica smiled warmly. "We've come a long way, and I'm excited to see where the journey takes us next."

As they celebrated, Alex felt a profound sense of gratitude and anticipation. The journey had been transformative, shaping him into the leader he was today. With the support of his friends, mentors, and the unwavering belief in their mission, he knew they were ready to face whatever challenges lay ahead.

As the evening drew to a close, Alex stood on the balcony, looking out over the city. The future was filled with uncertainty, but also with boundless potential. Embracing the future meant continuing to push the boundaries of medical science, inspiring the next generation of researchers, and making a lasting impact on global health.

With a sense of determination and hope, Alex turned back to join his friends, ready to embrace whatever the future held.

Chapter 30: The Journey Continues

The journey that Alex and his team had embarked on was far from over. The achievements they had celebrated were merely stepping stones on a path filled with potential. With each milestone, their vision for the future became clearer, and their commitment to advancing medical science grew stronger. The Global Neurological Research Network (GNRN) was thriving, and their global initiative was making a tangible difference in the lives of patients around the world.

One morning, as Alex was preparing for a lecture, he received a call from Dr. Vasquez. "Alex, I have some exciting news. Our research has been selected for a major funding grant from the International Medical Research Foundation. This grant will provide us with the resources to expand our clinical trials and reach even more patients."

Alex felt a surge of excitement. "That's incredible news, Dr. Vasquez. This funding will allow us to accelerate our progress and make an even greater impact."

The grant from the International Medical Research Foundation brought new opportunities and challenges. The team expanded their clinical trials, incorporating advanced technologies and innovative treatment protocols. The work was demanding, but the sense of purpose and the potential to change lives kept them motivated.

One evening, as Alex was reviewing the latest trial results, he received a call from Jessica. "Hey, Alex. I heard about the new funding. How are things going?"

"It's been intense, Jessica," Alex replied, "but incredibly rewarding. The new funding has opened up so many possibilities, and we're making real progress."

"You've always been determined, Alex," Jessica said, her voice filled with pride. "I'm so proud of everything you've accomplished."

The support from his friends continued to be a source of strength for

Alex. Emily, Sam, and Jessica remained steadfast in their encouragement, celebrating each milestone and offering words of wisdom.

As the months passed, the team's work continued to attract attention from the global medical community. Their innovative approaches and positive results were published in leading medical journals, and Alex was invited to speak at several high-profile conferences. The recognition and validation from his peers reinforced the importance of their mission and the impact of their collaborative efforts.

One day, while preparing for a presentation at an international medical symposium, Alex received a call from Dr. Harris. "Alex, I wanted to personally congratulate you on the progress you've made. Your work is truly groundbreaking, and I'm proud to see how far you've come."

"Thank you, Dr. Harris," Alex replied, feeling a deep sense of gratitude. "Your guidance and support have been invaluable throughout this journey."

The symposium was a resounding success, and Alex's presentation received widespread acclaim. The positive feedback and interest from the global medical community reinforced the importance of their work and the potential for future breakthroughs.

As the team returned to the institute, they were greeted with news that their research had been nominated for the prestigious Global Health Innovation Award. The nomination was a testament to their hard work and dedication, bringing a sense of pride and accomplishment to everyone involved.

Gathering with his friends to celebrate another milestone, Alex raised his glass in a toast. "To the journey that continues and the incredible path we've shared. We've faced many challenges, but we've also achieved so much. Here's to the future and the endless possibilities it holds."

"To the journey," Emily echoed, clinking her glass with his.

"And to the power of perseverance," Sam added.

Jessica smiled warmly. "We've come a long way, and I'm excited to see where the journey takes us next."

As they celebrated, Alex felt a profound sense of gratitude and anticipation. The journey had been transformative, shaping him into the leader he was today. With the support of his friends, mentors, and the unwavering belief in their mission, he knew they were ready to face whatever challenges lay ahead.

One evening, as Alex stood on the balcony, looking out over the city, he felt a deep sense of fulfillment. The future was filled with uncertainty, but also with boundless potential. Embracing the journey meant continuing to push the boundaries of medical science, inspiring the next generation of researchers, and making a lasting impact on global health.

With a sense of determination and hope, Alex turned back to join his friends, ready to embrace whatever the future held.

Chapter 31: A Legacy of Hope

The journey that Alex and his team had embarked on had been nothing short of extraordinary. The successes they had achieved, the challenges they had overcome, and the lives they had touched were all testaments to their unwavering dedication and commitment. As they approached the culmination of their work, Alex reflected on the legacy they were building—a legacy of hope and innovation in the field of neurology.

One morning, as Alex was reviewing the latest developments in their research, he received an unexpected call from Dr. Vasquez. "Alex, there's someone here to see you. I think you should come to my office."

Curious, Alex made his way to Dr. Vasquez's office. He found her standing with a young woman who looked both nervous and hopeful. "Alex, this is Sarah. She's a former patient who participated in our early trials."

Sarah smiled warmly, her eyes filled with gratitude. "Dr. Carter, I just wanted to thank you. Your research and the treatment I received have given me a second chance at life. I can now pursue my dreams and live without the constant fear of my illness."

Alex felt a wave of emotion. Moments like these reminded him of the real impact of their work. "Thank you, Sarah. Your strength and resilience are truly inspiring. I'm so glad to hear that you're doing well."

As Sarah left, Alex felt a renewed sense of purpose. The stories of patients like her were the driving force behind their research. They were not just working on treatments; they were restoring hope and transforming lives.

The team's efforts continued to gain recognition. The nomination for the Global Health Innovation Award turned into a win, and their work was celebrated at a prestigious ceremony attended by leaders from around the world. The recognition was a testament to their dedication and the impact of their research.

One evening, as Alex was preparing for another international conference, he received a call from his mother. "Alex, I saw the news about your award. Your father and I are so proud of you. You've accomplished so much."

"Thanks, Mom," Alex replied, his voice filled with emotion. "Your support has meant everything to me."

The conference was a resounding success, and Alex's presentation received widespread acclaim. The positive feedback and interest from the global medical community reinforced the importance of their work and the potential for future breakthroughs.

As the team returned to the institute, they were greeted with news that their research had led to the development of a new, groundbreaking treatment protocol. The protocol had shown exceptional results in clinical trials, offering new hope to patients with neurodegenerative diseases.

Gathering with his friends and colleagues to celebrate, Alex raised his glass in a toast. "To a legacy of hope and the incredible journey we've shared. We've faced many challenges, but we've also achieved so much. Here's to the future and the endless possibilities it holds."

"To hope and perseverance," Emily echoed, clinking her glass with his.

"And to the power of innovation," Sam added.

Jessica smiled warmly. "We've come a long way, and I'm excited to see where the journey takes us next."

As they celebrated, Alex felt a profound sense of gratitude and anticipation. The journey had been transformative, shaping him into the leader he was today. With the support of his friends, mentors, and the unwavering belief in their mission, he knew they were ready to face whatever challenges lay ahead.

One evening, as Alex stood on the balcony, looking out over the city, he felt a deep sense of fulfillment. The future was filled with uncertainty, but also with boundless potential. Embracing the future meant continuing to push the boundaries of medical science, inspiring the next generation of researchers, and making a lasting impact on global health.

With a sense of determination and hope, Alex turned back to join his friends, ready to embrace whatever the future held.

www.ingramcontent.com/pod-product-compliance
Lightning Source LLC
Chambersburg PA
CBHW071940210526
45479CB00002B/753